LOVE
YOURSELF
HEALTHY

A Physician's Guide to Healing MS

Dear
Rosemary
To your best
health!
Love Cynthia
2/1/17

CYNTHIA GUY, MD

Dedication

I dedicate this book to my loving husband, who always encouraged me to follow my dreams. Because of his support, I applied to medical school as a second career and flourished in my medical practice while he helped take care of our girls. I love you very much, Stuart, and wish you many more years of health.

Acknowledgments

I gratefully acknowledge all of the physician and non-physician experts who have guided me in my journey for more—more learning, more health, and more vitality. Doctors Tom O'Brian, Perlmutter, Wahls, and Mercola, thank you for sharing your cutting-edge nutrition and health principles with me and the rest of the public. David Wolfe—you are awesome. It's an honor to be your student.

I would also like to acknowledge my daughter Laura and her help in writing and editing this book. I could not have completed this project without her.

Thank you to my daughter Michelle who always encouraged me with this project.

Contents

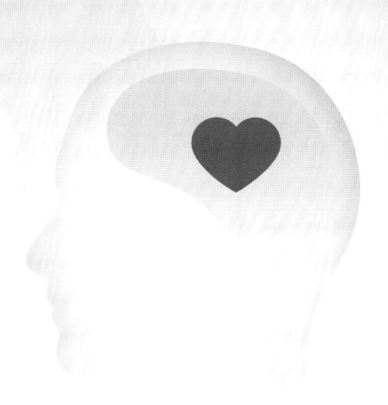

INTRODUCTION
Your MS
Diagnosis: Day 1

Being diagnosed with MS, or multiple sclerosis, is one of the scariest things that ever happened to me. If you have just been diagnosed, you probably have a lot of questions, doubts, and anxieties. Some of these concerns have answers, and some do not.

You see, multiple sclerosis is not a disease that has many answers. To modern medicine, this progressive ailment can only be managed— and not very successfully. Immediately after your diagnosis, you are told that there is no cure and that this is something that you may have to face alone and need to manage for the rest of your life.

The prognosis does not look good for the average person that is diagnosed. Treatments are limited and invasive, and times ahead will be challenging. At least, this is what I was told when I was first diagnosed back in the '90s.

For better or worse, I was also a doctor. Being a doctor, I was able to experience that unique moment in medicine when every part of me rejected my prognosis, and I remained in denial for a number of years. I could not accept that I was doomed to exist with this disease for the rest of my life. I had to take action!

Eventually, I started to seek answers to improve the gloomy outcome of my prognosis. This set me on a journey that helped me change my disease process and my life. I found real ways to deal with multiple sclerosis and began to understand just how flawed current treatment of this disease is for many in the Western world.

Day 1 is a hard day to get through, but I have good news for you. What your doctor has told you is not the beginning and the end of your options. This book will walk you through all of the excellent research and personal insight that helped and continues to help me reduce and manage my MS successfully.

Inside you will find techniques, tips, and cutting-edge information that will inspire and motivate you to deal with your MS head on. This book encapsulates all of the medical research I have studied as well as my own personal experiences and insights in enhancing my quality of life. My greatest wish is to pass this information on to you so that you can learn how to make your own life easier and live more comfortably with MS.

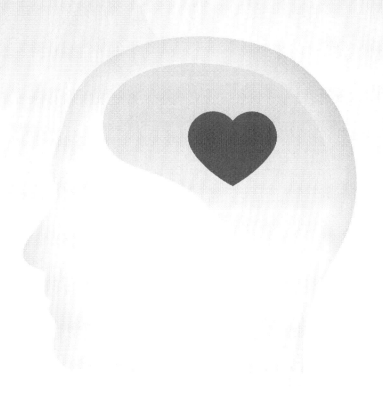

CHAPTER **1**

My Journey With MS

"Oddly enough, MS has made my life so much better than it was before. I now appreciate what I have and I am not running around like a rat in a maze."

TERI GARR

Most people that are diagnosed with MS have to go through a long and arduous testing process to be diagnosed. Then, at the end, you are sat down and told that you have multiple sclerosis and that there is no cure—and that maybe some drugs can help you along the way.

Before my diagnosis, I was a very successful physician at the tipping point of my medical career. Then it all changed.

At 33 years old, I decided to pursue my goal of becoming a physician and entered medical school. At the time, I was a qualified nurse anesthetist with a hunger to complete my medical degree.

I have always been a very goal-oriented person. Once I had secured my doctorate, my husband, kids, and I immigrated to the United States in search of greener pastures. My dream was to practice medicine in the land of opportunity.

I trained as an anesthesiologist at a major tertiary hospital in St Louis, Missouri. Slowly, I worked my way up, eventually becoming

Chief of Anesthesiology at Missouri Baptist Medical Center and overseeing a staff of 42 people.

Once I had reached the top of my field, I harnessed my skills as a medical entrepreneur and established the first independent pain center in St Louis. Truly, my family and I seized on the American dream, and we lived it.

Those days were hard, long, and grueling. I scarcely remember a time when I was not working at three times the pace of other people. For many years, I was driven to achieve; I wanted it all, and there was a price to pay for that.

The Trouble With Symptoms

As I got older, I began to notice some symptoms that I initially confused with age: things like fatigue, balance problems, and vision issues can very easily be chalked up to "getting older." Unlike many other MS sufferers, I was not diagnosed between the ages of 20 and 40.

The stress of achievement had finally taken its toll, and my body was reacting in ways that were not consistent with your "average" age concerns. For example, I started to drop things frequently; I started to stumble with my left leg; I experienced unrelenting fatigue and numbness and tingling in my feet. I was actually told by one of my physician colleagues that I was a post-menopausal over-achiever who needed to retire.

Of course—and any MS sufferer will tell you this—the road to identifying that your symptoms could be MS is a long one. Most of the time you will have to sit through multiple appointments getting pathology (blood) tests done, and they will all turn up clear. You will check your thyroid, your liver, your kidneys—everything.

For me, nothing explained the strange sensations in my legs and hands. I knew something was wrong, and I was perpetually fatigued. I remember calling my husband to drive me home in the middle of the day because I was too tired to drive home. Once the blood tests turn up clean, you are sent off for a host of other tests—scans, MRIs, and, eventually, neurology.

Most neurologists can diagnose MS, but so many factors have to be in place to make an accurate diagnosis. It is not uncommon for people to be declared fine only to return with the same symptoms or worse that prompt further investigation.

In my case, one neurologist initially diagnosed me with carpal tunnel syndrome and told me I did not have MS. At the time, I was happy to hear that. But my accidentally stumbling with my left foot continued—one night resulting in a fall—so I decided to seek another opinion.

No one with MS has the same symptoms. It is really like a crap shoot; you never know what you are going to get. But as a doctor, I knew that my symptoms were real enough to cause alarm—so I searched for answers until one presented itself.

My Multiple Sclerosis Diagnosis

The second opinion I received was not one I was prepared for or even entertained. I was diagnosed with multiple sclerosis at age 60. My doctor stated he had good news and bad news—that I did not have a brain tumor but that I did have MS. It was the year 2000, and I had already been experiencing symptoms since 1995. Although I was once extremely active, spinning every day and walking, I would attribute the stu Terri Garr mbling and tight muscles to other things—but never MS.

In the car after the appointment, my husband started crying.

It forced me to retire and sell my practice, which was the hardest thing I ever had to do as an adult because I could not imagine what I would do with my life. What does a workaholic do when she stops working? I would often schedule in more than 20 patients a day, but my fatigue had grown so bad that I could barely function and had to start rescheduling appointments. Sometimes I would be too tired to drive home and had to call my husband.

Letting go of achievement is something no one prepares you for, and as an over-achiever, it left a gaping hole in my life. Maybe I will just de-escalate my practice into something less stressful, I thought. I started to do clinical research and started a weight management practice.

For several years I kept busy working, albeit to a lesser degree than as an anesthesiologist, but I still did not focus on taking care of myself and working to heal my MS. It took me many years to really focus on healing.

Being a doctor, I knew that I would have to employ all of my research ability and tenacity to find answers that greater minds than mine could not see. The establishment was telling me that MS would consume my life, but I could not believe that.

Quality of life is all that you have when you get older. It is hard enough trying to live comfortably without a disease process robbing you of peace during your average day. I felt that voice inside me rage.

It took me years to accept my diagnosis. Looking back, I think this was a function of both my own ego and the fact that I was in the Relapsing and Remitting stage of MS. Symptoms came and went; one day I felt normal and the next I experienced a number of symptoms, such as numbness and tingling. As a result, it took me years to take action and years to look for solutions.

If I think about it now, it is amazing to me that no other alternatives were given other than "retire" and "you are working too much." I had MRI studies done, but they were inconclusive. I repeated these five years later as things got worse. All that time I could have helped myself if I had realized the extent of this disease. I sold my practice to the Washington University of Medicine (my alma mater) and went for more tests. The later MRIs proved, finally, that my MS diagnosis was irrefutable.

So what if modern medicine could not tell me the answers? I knew they were out there. I decided to start looking and to not give up until I had restored my own health!

My doctor did not make it any easier by recommending modern treatments involving drugs and surgeries. Even though some drugs may modify the disease progression, they never really eliminate it, and they do not necessarily make you healthier due to secondary effects and adverse reactions. I took medication for almost five years and was eventually told to stop them when my disease worsened. At one stage my doctor said I would be confined to a bed for months if I did not improve. They told me to seek out support groups and begin with immune-suppressant drugs.

Part of my journey would be discovering this the hard way. I had to come up with a game plan. I was still working the lecture circuits and doing clinical research; my kids were establishing themselves professionally, and I still wanted to travel. I did not accept that I would be confined to a bed.

I want to share my findings with you in this book so that you can also find some peace and health among the MS chaos.

The Physical Consequences of MS

As I mentioned, there are lots of consequences involved in having MS. Some of these are physical, some are psychological, and more still are emotional. No MS sufferer can know exactly what their MS will do; it is a very unpredictable disease.

Both sets of consequences differ from patient to patient. I experienced an inability to raise my left leg, which caused foot drop, and I had severe fatigue. I was also working through levels of depression and denial. I believe it was the denial that prompted me to accept the medicine that the doctors prescribed, injecting myself daily. From what I read, the medication would arrest the disease's progression. I had no "serious" adverse reaction, but my

MS symptoms did not improve. I gained weight as well, which made things harder.

Then I developed lipodystrophy in my injection site. This is when your fat disappears from a place in your body. It's unsightly, looks like holes. I had to inject my medication into what I called "gutters" in my abdomen. I asked my neurologist what was happening, stating that if this was occurring at a superficial level, what was happening on a cellular level. She said she did not know. That was when I decided to stop the drugs. If my neurologist did not know what the chemicals were doing to my cells on a molecular level, then I did not want to risk any more damage. I took this drug, Copaxone, for four years.

The physical consequences of MS can manifest for you in a number of ways. These are the signs and symptoms that are most common in MS sufferers:

- *Strange, "out of the norm" sensations.* Many people that have developed MS notice it because of strange itching, burning, numbness, stabbing, or tearing pain in their body. Pins and needles are most common in the limbs.

- *Difficulty walking.* People with MS often struggle to walk because they struggle with muscle pain, spasms, and weakness. Things like numb feet and widespread balance problems can also make walking harder.

- *Muscle spasms.* These occur mainly in the legs, and they can range from mild to powerfully painful spasms. Some 40%[1] of people believe that these are an early symptom of MS.

- *Speech and talking.* When MS gets really bad, it causes speech disturbances like slurring, nasal speech, or pausing for long periods between words. Swallowing can also become problematic in late stages of MS.

---

1   Recognize Multiple Sclerosis Symptoms, http://www.webmd.com/multiple-sclerosis/guide/multiple-sclerosis-diagnosis

- *Dizziness is a real MS concern.* Sufferers with MS often feel exceptionally dizzy or lightheaded, to the point where they have to stay in bed to make it go away.

- *Bladder and bowel trouble.* Some 80% of MS patients[2] have trouble with their bladders or bowels. Whether it is constipation, needing to go all the time, or not feeling like you have gone, these are persistent problems.

MS can affect the human body in so many ways from your brain, vision, tongue, heart, immune system, and lungs to your reproductive system, bowel, bladder, bones, limbs, and movement.

The Psychological Consequences of MS

Along with the many, many physical consequences of having MS, there are some pretty prominent psychological ones as well. It is important to note that many medications that you can take for MS do aggravate already fragile psychological states.

- *Depression is common with MS.* Along with the constant attack on your central nervous system, people with MS find that being depressed is part of the package. Loss of energy, sadness, and feelings of hopelessness are precursors.

- *Anxiety is a huge MS symptom.* People with MS often complain of high stress lifestyles and crushing anxiety because of their disease and the demands it makes on their life. Stress can lead to all sorts of tertiary health concerns.

- *Cognitive dysfunction with MS.* Some studies indicate that 43– 65%[3] of diagnosed MS sufferers have some kind of cognitive impairment on neuropsychological tests. Slowed thought

---

2   Multiple Sclerosis and Bladder Control Problems, http://www.webmd.com/multiple-sclerosis/guide/bladder-control-problems

3   Stefanie Hoffman, Marc Tittgemeyer, D Yves von Cramon, Cognitive Impairment in Multiple Sclerosis, www.researchgate.net/...Cognitive_impairment...multiple_s...

processing speeds, problems with verbal and visual memory, issues with attention and concentration, and verbal fluency can be affected.

Along with these come many smaller concerns that can cause mental distress, which compound on things like limited mobility and sexual dysfunction. It is incredibly important for an MS sufferer to have support when they are diagnosed.

Many of the psychological consequences of MS can be treated in supportive environments. These must be taken seriously, as the incidence of suicide among MS patients is high. Some 15% of all MS deaths[4] are suicide related, with depression and anxiety being culprits.

For MS patients with central nervous system damage, using drugs and alcohol is especially damaging, further aggravating the neurological damage that exists there.

The Emotional Consequences of MS

Along with physical and psychological consequences, there are also emotional consequences for having MS. These responses can be profound depending on the unpredictable nature of the disease.

In addition to the emotional reactions from having this disease, the demyelination and nerve fiber damage in the brain can also cause emotional changes. Then there are the dozens of medications than directly impact your emotional state.

- *Severe depressive episodes and lesser depressive episodes.* A few hours of feeling down for no reason can sometimes become weeks of very real depression that you may not have experienced before.

---

4   Ida S Haussleiter, Martin Brune, Georg Juckel, Psychopathology in Multiple Sclerosis, http://www.ncbi.nlm.nih.gov/pmc/articles/PMC3002616/

- *Generalized distress and anxiety responses are common in patients with MS.* But these also cause rapid mood swings and emotional liability. Often the mood is not directly related to any exterior cause but arises from nowhere.
- *Some MS patients find that they have pseudo bulbar affects,* which cause uncontrollable laughing or crying. These can occur during a particularly bad attack that lasts for some weeks.
- *Emotional instability caused by MS* can also lead to inappropriate sexual behavior and aggressiveness.

Of the many challenges that people face when being diagnosed with MS, the emotional challenges are the worst. Every new ache and pain triggers distress that affects sufferers on so many levels. That is why it is critical for patients with MS to seek support and care.

There are many roads that MS sufferers can walk down, and many of them may lead to worsening symptoms. I personally believe that through trial and error, many of the emotional symptoms of MS can be alleviated by alternative treatments.

Traditional, Conventional Therapies: The Long Road

There is no cure for MS, as I mentioned earlier, although there are a wide variety of conventional treatments that can slow the progression of the disease and treat the relapses or "attacks" that keep happening.

- Disease-modifying drugs can be taken daily to prevent attacks, although they come with a host of side effects that eventually leave you worse off than before.
- Deep brain stimulation is a surgical procedure that can help control tremors, but it comes with a number of risks.
- Medications can be taken to control muscle spasms and stiffness, but again, these are loaded with side effects that will not make you healthier in the long run.

- Physiotherapy can be used to facilitate flexibility in troublesome legs, and it helps to keep limbs performing at their best.

The main issue that I had with conventional treatment is the same one you may have. Drugs cannot be taken indefinitely, or they will seriously damage your internal organs and result in secondary and tertiary disease.

Surgery is so invasive, and with the risks, it is just not worth it. So the choices that your doctor gives you are to be cut open or to be drugged. I have always seen the value in medication, but long term, of course, it carries its risks.

The bottom line is that conventional treatment is a long road for which you need to consider the pros and cons due to mostly questionable outcomes. You will try different medications, suffer with different side effects, and may end up worse off for it. Then you might resort to surgery, and your quality of life could eventually deteriorate.

The Only Answer That Matters: Quality of Life with MS

With all of the physical, mental, and emotional consequences I was facing, conventional treatments did not work for me. I was not offered any alternative medication for Secondary Progressive MS—only for Relapsing and Remitting.

I could let my disease run rampant, or I could search for a better alternative. I turned to the only answer that matters—quality of life. How could I obtain quality of life with MS? How could I minimize the symptoms and improve my quality of life?

You will end up asking these same questions, and they will be tough to find answers for. I explored every nook and cranny for you, and this is what I discovered. *Doctors have been downplaying the importance of nutrition, stress management, and exercise for too long.*

With the right balance of nutrition, exercise, stress management, and alternative treatments, I managed to completely pull myself back from the brink of being close to bedridden from MS. The results, in my mind, do not lie. They are an absolute revelation.

The moment I realized my "alternative" treatments were working, I wanted to tell the world. Why do doctors not tell their patients about them? Why were drugs the only options I was given? The medical establishment needs to consider new and healthier therapies.

Like me, you will find that the solutions in this book are too simple to be true. I thought so. The thing is, they are true—and they work. Not only that, but they work without harming your body and without causing internal organ damage or adverse reactions.

I am sure you will agree that the options offered here are simple, cost-effective, and relatively easy to implement. Quality of life is at your doorstep. What is required is for you to be motivated to follow the guidelines in this book. I am confident that if I can change my situation in my late 60s, you can change yours also. Do yourself a favor, and try these methods first. If they do not work, then continue to search for ones that do. But if they do work, you would have just saved your own life. And that is worth fighting for. I decided to help myself and began reading. It led me to nutrition, and my friend, Betty Berger, suggested I try the Kushi Institute and go on a macrobiotic diet.

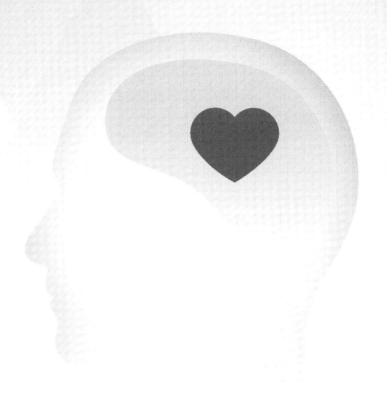

CHAPTER 2

Multiple Sclerosis in Society

"Currently, there is no cure for MS, but there are treatments that modify disease activity, slow the course of the disease, and alleviate its effects."

NANCY J. HOLLAND

Now that you know my story and how I came to be so inspired to conduct lengthy research into alternative therapies, I want to give you some solid grounding in what MS is all about and what you can expect after diagnosis.

Part of the anxiety about MS is the fear that you will contract all the symptoms, and this is just not true. Everyone is different—and I fervently believe that everyone can benefit from alternative therapies in some meaningful way.

The rise of autoimmune diseases is an amazing thing to me. My own diagnosis was not the norm—I was not the typical Caucasian female living in the North, and I was diagnosed at 60, not 40 or less. This made me wonder if there was not some other trigger that made my immune system go haywire. One of my theories involves stress as a trigger, but nutrition and exercise are definitely factors.

What Is Multiple Sclerosis?

If you were anything like me, you barely caught what your doctor was saying to you when you were diagnosed. The information came in a blur, and you could not understand any of it, such was the shock.

To recap, multiple sclerosis is an immune-mediated process where your immune system has an abnormal response to your central nervous system. The CNS is made up of your brain, spinal cord, and optic nerve.

While not quite an autoimmune disease, MS is certainly considered an immune-mediated one; the only problem is that science has yet to discover why your body targets certain immune cells and not others.

Inside your central nervous system, your immune system attacks myelin, or that fatty substance that surrounds and insulates nerve fibers, until they attack the nerve fibers themselves.

When myelin becomes damaged, it creates scar tissue over your nerves known as sclerosis, which is where the name comes from. People with this disease literally have multiple sites on their body where myelin has been damaged, causing the symptoms.

The Rise of Autoimmune Diseases

When your own body turns on you, it is an alarming situation to face. Yet millions of people all over the Western world face autoimmune diseases every day. There has been a massive boom in these diseases over the last 50 years, leading us to ask the question—why?

With diabetes, celiac disease, asthma, and MS on a rapid upturn, there are now more than 50 million Americans affected by these diseases, according to American Autoimmune Related Diseases Association Inc.[5]

There are many theories about why your body's own security team would attack itself. One of the most interesting I have come across is from Dr. Fasano, who discovered that three factors were prevalent in the diagnosis of almost all autoimmune diseases.

The three factors were a genetic predisposition, an environmental

---

5   Autoimmune Statistics, http://www.aarda.org/autoimmune-information/autoimmune-statistics/

factor (like an infection), and a leaky gut. His research indicated that the presence of a leaky gut caused the environmental factors to trigger the genetic predisposition.

When there is excess zonulin (zonulin is a protein that modulates how permeable the cells are in your digestive tract) in your gut, it opens the door for viruses and bacteria and all sorts of chemicals and parasites to enter your blood stream. In response, your body creates lots of T cells to deal with the invaders.

When your T cells (T cells are a type of lymphocyte that are important to cell immunity) are at high levels all the time, this is what causes an autoimmune disease. The good news, however, is that a healthy diet helps your body once again seal that leaky barrel, which greatly reduces autoimmunity.

This could be the reason why I have had such incredible results by changing my diet and eating for life in addition to implementing exercise and stress management. I am going to share my experiences and methods with you later on in this book.

The History of Multiple Sclerosis

In the year 2000, I began my MS research. I had already decided that weight was important because I was having so much trouble walking, even while using a cane. As the disease progressed, I stopped using drugs as it did not cause my disease to "burn out" as I was told it would.

Multiple sclerosis was first spotted in autopsy reports dating back to 1838.[6] The reports went into detail about the plaques or expanses of scar tissue caused by inflammation of the brain.

Then, in 1869, Jean-Martin Charcot—a French professor—made an association between autopsy plaques with a deceased woman, who had tremors, strange eye movements, and slurred speech. The lesions, he deduced, corresponded with the symptoms.

---

6   Erica Roth, The History of Multiple Sclerosis: How Far Have We Come?, http://www.healthline.com/health-slideshow/history-multiple-sclerosis-how-far-have-we-come

It was not until 1870 that MS was recognized officially. Two doctors, one from England and one from New York, observed a large range of neurological symptoms in their female patients.

Later on, in 1930, there was a massive incline in medical breakthroughs because of more modern technology. The medical profession began to study the progression and widespread symptoms of the disease.

By 1935 Dr. Thomas Rivers proved his theory with lab animals—that MS was not a viral ailment but an immune system disease. With that revelation came the formation of the National Multiple Sclerosis Society.

By 1960 doctors established that it was myelin that was being attacked by the body's immune system, giving rise to its designation as an autoimmune disease. The 1980s brought about the MRI, which proved the damage being done inside patients.

Then—with 1990s and modern drug technology—treatments were developed to help manage and reduce the damage done by multiple sclerosis. When the 2000s hit, it was discovered that vitamin D has a protective effect against genetic MS.

These days, new discoveries are happening all the time. For example, it was discovered in 2011 that 60–80%[7] of people with MS experience heat sensitivity. Only time will tell if medical science can come up with a cure. Until then, it is up to you to heal your own MS.

Traditional Testing for the Disease

Traditional testing for MS is not an easy process. In fact, it is so difficult that it can take years to reach a final verdict from a neurologist. Modern medicine uses a process of elimination to make sure that it is not anything else first.

---

7   Cooling Program Helps People With MS Cope With Heat Intolerance, http://www. advancesinms.ca/article/cooling-program-helps-people-with-ms-cope-with-heat-intolerance/

- You will spend a lot of time doing blood tests and various other kinds of tests to rule out basic dysfunctions that could indicate other diseases or conditions are to blame.

- It is very important to get a diagnosis as soon as possible because the brain and spinal damage that occurs can be slowed and treated—the sooner the better.

- If you have suffered from an episode of optic neuritis, there are now tests that can check the condition of your optic nerve. They are painless and use an imaging tool to check out the condition of your myelin. Studies show that MS sufferers' optic nerve always looks different from other people's, which means it is important to diagnose.

- The doctor must perform investigations and meet certain criteria for diagnosing MS. There must be evidence of damage in at least two areas of your central nervous system. They must also rule out *all* other possible diagnoses and find evidence that damage occurred at two different points in time.

Invasive and non-invasive tests are used, including pathology, medical history compilation, magnetic resonance imaging, cerebrospinal fluid, evoked potentials, MRI scans, neurological examinations, and lumbar punctures.

It is important to note that there is no one test or one finding that can confirm that you have MS for certain. Sometimes MS is misdiagnosed and could be a number of other things. I would suggest getting a second and a third opinion.

Your Complicated Diagnosis: MS

Just like MS itself, individuals have different diagnostic journeys to get their diagnosis. You or your loved one perhaps went straight to the MRI and other cleaner methods because of strong symptoms. Someone else might have spent two to four years going to hospitals, doctors, and specialists to find out what these strange, recurring symptoms were.

The truth is that even though a multiple sclerosis diagnostic is difficult, they are fairly accurate. The scarring that forms from myelin damage is highly visible on an MRI scan, although some 5%[8] of people with MS do not show damage there.

If your MRI scan does not work, it is likely that you will be asked to do a lumbar puncture, which is a much more invasive procedure. Your cerebrospinal fluid will be extracted and sent off for analysis. This is only necessary if your MRI is inconclusive.

MS will show up in this test because 95% of people[9] with MS show oligoclonal brands, which refers to the presence of immunoglobulin. These proteins are carried in white blood cells and can indicate inflammation of your central nervous system.

If neither of those work—or before being told to have an MRI— you may need to undergo evoked potentials or an EP test. In MS, it is called a visual evoked potential, and all it does is measure the messages sent from your eyes to your central nervous system.

Whether you have had a quick diagnosis shock or a long slog through eliminating all other potential causes, arriving at an MS diagnosis is bad news. Treatment for your MS will be just as hard and tricky, with different people responding to different things.

In 2004 I focused my research on nutrition. I learned how to be macrobiotic for a number of years and then discovered the qualities of raw food. I even took courses with David Wolfe and learned to be a raw foodist, although it was massively challenging to stick to the diet.

On a combination of both diets, I lost 40 pounds. I ate macro and raw food, and for the first time, experienced the benefits of

---

8   Magnetic Resonance Imaging, http://www.nationalmssociety.org/Symptoms-Diagnosis/Diagnosing-Tools/MRI

9   Diagnosis, http://www.mstrust.org.uk/information/publications/msexplained/diagnosis.jsp

focusing on nutritional healing. I could walk around without a cane, and my fatigue had gone away enough that I could do more in my day. From 2004, with 10 years of nutritional focus, I felt inspired to share the benefits of nutrition with others. Becoming gluten free and incorporating the ketogenic diet has given me even greater wellbeing.

I would encourage you to try the alternative route first before handing yourself over to a lifetime of drugs, hospital visits, and medical expenses. As a doctor, it pains me to say this, but pursuing alternative therapy—after trying conventional therapies first—was the best thing that I ever did.

MS in Western Society and Around the World

Typically, multiple sclerosis is handled by Western civilization as a chronic and degenerative disease with poor prognosis. While medications do work to a certain extent, one must remember that the profile of serious or adverse events exists with most drugs.

And that is why I became hesitant to continue drug therapy. After four and a half years of taking daily injections, I did not see any improvement.

Long-term drug treatments can lead to kidney and liver damage, and these are not additional issues that you want. Some people will refuse conventional drug therapy but then use over-the-counter medication such as painkillers and anti-inflammatories that can equally cause ill-effects. Fortunately, there is also a growing body of evidence that suggests natural treatments and alternative therapies can help many MS sufferers. I am inclined to believe that natural healing is far more beneficial for you based on my own experience taking immuno-modulators and then moving over to more natural treatments. All over the globe, people with MS are deciding that dealing with the disease means taking action, not ingesting a pill or going in for a procedure.

To me, that is encouraging. Multiple sclerosis can be life changing because most of the people diagnosed with it are still young. My hope is that your youth does not cloud your judgment and that you do not blindly follow the treatment plan of one doctor without exploring the alternatives.

The Latest Research on MS

The latest research on MS is controversial to say the least, but science does not lie. I have included some of the latest findings that you should know about here. But it is up to you to continue to do this for yourself as the years roll by.

- The latest research from the American Society for Microbiology suggests that an airborne food toxin called epsilon may be the environmental trigger for MS,[10] as their animal studies have concluded.
- Evidence suggests that medical marijuana in the form of pills or spray can ease patient problems with MS-related spasticity, pain, and urination concerns. This from the American Academy of Neurology, as recently as March 2014.[11]
- The University of Pittsburgh,[12] School of Health Sciences, found that stem cells from human muscle tissue can repair nerve damage and restore function in mice that have sciatic nerve injuries.

---

10   Bacterial Toxin Potential Trigger for Multiple Sclerosis, http://www.sciencedaily.com/releases/2014/01/140128153940.htm

11   Medical Marijuana May Ease Some MS; Little Evidence for Other Complementary or Alternative Therapies, http://www.sciencedaily.com/releases/2014/03/140324181258.htm

12   Stem Cells From Muscle Can Repair Nerve Damage After Injury, http://www.sciencedaily.com/releases/2014/03/140318190035.htm

- The University of Copenhagen[13] recently announced that new blood cells fight brain inflammation. Hyperactivity of immune cells called T cells induces chronic inflammation and degeneration in the brain; this new type of blood cell can combat this in MS patients.
- The Kessler Foundation[14] discovered that people with tertiary level education or higher level education are at a much reduced risk for cognitive impairment from MS. This suggests continuous learning could be a preventative measure.

These are just some of the excellent studies that are being performed in medicine right now to find a cure for MS. Being aware of new research will keep you looking for opportunities to relieve and heal your MS.

Population Reports and Societal Impact

Because multiple sclerosis is the number one cause of disability among young people, it has a huge impact on Western society and costs the medical establishment billions of dollars every year. This is a concern as the prevalence of the disease is global.

- The prevalence of MS is estimated to be 30 out of every 100,000[15] people.
- Europe has the greatest prevalence (80 per 100,000), then Eastern Mediterranean (14.9), and America (8.3).
- There are almost no cases of MS among lower income countries, with the highest prevalence of MS estimated among high income countries.

---

13   New Blood Cells Fight Brain Inflammation, http://news.ku.dk/all_news/2014/02/blood_cells_fight_brain_inflammation/

14   Cognition, http://www.ms-uk.org/cognition

15   Atlas, http://www.who.int/mental_health/neurology/Atlas_MS_WEB.pdf (all data points)

- The World Health Organization estimates that there are some 1.3 million people right now that are suffering with MS in the world.

- The average onset of MS starts at 29.2 years of age. There are MS groups and support centers all over the globe, with a 73.2% prevalence.

- MS is uncommon in Japan, China, and South America. It is non-existent with the Lapp people of Scandinavia. Native Americans also very rarely contract the disease.

- MS is most prevalent in Caucasian communities, especially among first degree relatives. In twins, a 30% concordance rate is estimated.[16]

- Females contract MS a lot more often than males do with a 3:1 ratio in certain cases.

Learning more about the relationship between what you eat and your immune system is critical for MS patients. Gut health is the key—meaning that if your gut is not happy, it may trigger an autoimmune process that causes many diseases. It also causes brain fog, depression, fatigue, and many other concerns for an MS patient. "Gut health first" needs to become your new mantra!

I was addicted to gluten and everything with gluten in it. Once I had cut that out—and it was hard—my health changed. I was 60 years old, and I had to change my eating habits. Since performing all of the nutritional changes, I am pleased to report that my health has improved by 70–75%. If I had continued taking modern medicine, I would be bed-ridden. If I had to portion it down now, I would say stress was a major factor, and removing sugar and gluten from my diet was the best thing I ever did. Being surrounded by positive people was also important.

---

16   Multiple Sclerosis Susceptibility to; MS, http://omim.org/entry/126200

Multiple sclerosis is clearly a global disease, but it mainly impacts the Western world. Scientists simply do not understand why some peoples and some places seem to have no MS incidence. Further study will have to clear up those questions as we evolve.

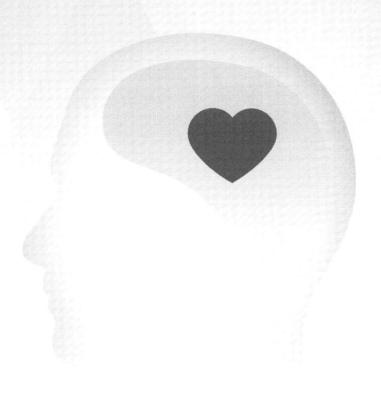

CHAPTER **3**

Research on the Symptoms of MS

"There are only two ways to live your life. One is as though nothing is a miracle. The other is as though everything is a miracle."

ALBERT EINSTEIN

Multiple sclerosis comes on slowly. For most people, they do not even realize that something is wrong until their second or third attack. The very first episode is called the "clinical isolated syndrome," which occurs between the ages of 20 and 40.

The moment the second attack happens, it is considered to be relapsing and remitting multiple sclerosis. If the disease progresses from the very beginning, it is an alarming race to immobility, pain, and disability. I did not pursue additional therapy after my four-year long experience with Copaxone and the missing fat gullies in my stomach. It was a decidedly excellent choice.

Investigating Chronic Fatigue

It is true that 80%[17] of people with MS will suffer with chronic fatigue at some point. This is not a great stat, especially if you are diagnosed at a young age.

---

17 Multiple Sclerosis and Fatigue, http://www.webmd.com/multiple-sclerosis/guide/ms-related-fatigue

For MS sufferers, fatigue is not the same as being tired. It is like spending 18 hours on a plane, switching between three trains, and not sleeping for two days. Every single day, some people with MS go to sleep fatigued and wake up fatigued.

No amount of sleep combats it—it is relentless tiredness that does not let up. Sometimes it lasts for a week, sometimes a month. It could even be chronic. Fatigue from MS is the single most horrible thing about the disease because it saps the life right out of you.

The latest research indicates that changes to heat and cold as well as stress can set off a fatigue attack. The same can be said for viruses or bacterial infections. When you do suffer from a fatigue attack, the best thing to do is to avoid physical exertion and to rest. When I started to experience fatigue, I began to coordinate my work schedule to do the most challenging medical procedures in the morning before I got tired in the afternoon. If I had a late meeting, I made sure to nap at least a half hour beforehand.

In a recent MS focus poll, 89%[18] of MS sufferers said that fatigue had a major impact on their quality of life. The interesting thing is that a lot of MS people are not your average lazy sorts, so they get a lot done, even though it hurts them.

Your job is to learn to recognize fatigue when it strikes, manage it, and prepare your days so that you do not encounter an accident.

Focusing in on Physical Numbness

Another multiple sclerosis symptom that is very common is numbness. This is often described as a strange sensation to begin with because it can be so mild. But numbness in your limbs can be mild or severe, sometimes leaving your legs immovable.

MS sufferers deal with numb faces, numb arms and legs, and even numbness on their body. This can cause difficulty holding things, walking, and a host of other concerns. Numbness of the hands

18   Alison Potts, It's Like Being Switched Off, http://www.bbc.com/news/health-18207490

especially can result in dropping objects and perhaps injury.

When I was first diagnosed, I used to drop objects like cups and pens due to left hand weakness. I also began to lose dexterity in my right hand and lost fine motor skills. To this day, I cannot button my blouse or put on an earring, and my handwriting is terrible.

At first the numbness may not be that concerning, but it puts you in danger. This is because the modern household is full of heat sources that can harm you if you are not careful.

Let's get something straight—nothing cures numbness. It feels horrible and can cause havoc in your life, but most of the time it recedes on its own. You can choose to go to your neurologist, but they will just inject you with a temporary fix, and they are not great for you.

Numbness is also part of tingling, burning, and that "pins and needles" feeling, which I will explore below. The best treatment available for numbness is stretching. Stretching relaxes the nerves that innervate the muscles, thereby decreasing the spasticity that causes numbness. Relaxation exercises using breathing techniques are quite helpful.

Those Tingles and Pins and Needles

While we are on the topic of numbness, there are three main types that you should know about. It is very rare to experience anesthesia, which is complete loss of feeling in one area. That said, you should have it checked out if that is the case.

- *Paresthesia* is what you call those pins and needles or those tingling, buzzing, and crawling sensations that you get all over the place. They do not hurt, but they can irritate you to the point of distress.
- *Dysesthesia* is when there is a burning sensation along your nerve. When this happens, touch and pressure sensations change and normal contact becomes extremely painful.

- *Hyperpathia* is when you have an increased sensitivity to pain. Press anywhere on your body, and if this is happening, it will hurt.

As I mentioned, these are more irritating than painful—but they can also be creepy, alarming, and terrifying if they escalate in ways you are not prepared for.

When the tingling first started, I used to think, "The ants are back." I felt them on my back and shoulders intermittently, which made me anxious, mostly because I did not know what was happening or where these feelings were coming from. Today I still have tingling, and my feet burn sometimes; I cope by stretching, which helps release the sensations. I also take all-natural, anti-inflammatory supplements, which I will talk about in later chapters.

If you experience numbness or any of these sensations during an MS attack, they will end when the attack passes. There is usually no need for medication, just caution.

When Nothing Seems to Balance

Being off balance and dizzy and having trouble walking in the right direction are all part of the experience of living with MS. Like most symptoms, everyone experiences different levels of dizziness. Some cannot get out of bed; others simply find walking a challenge.

Stumbling was one of the first MS symptoms I experienced. In the beginning, I thought I was wearing the wrong shoes, so I bought and changed shoes all the time until I finally accepted the fact that I had a drop foot, which caused me to lose balance.

There are lots of reasons why you are getting dizzy and off balance as a person with MS. Your central nervous system works on all three parts of your balance process: input, processing, and output. That means your brain will send overdue, misleading, or incomplete information to your limbs, which seriously makes movement a challenge. Your inputs for balance are your ears, your vision, and your other senses.

Having visual problems, inner ear issues, and numbness will interrupt the messages that your brain is trying to send to your limbs. Nerve damage in the cerebellum or brainstem can cause bad nausea and troublesome vertigo.

Finally, and the worst one I think, are the outputs. What happens to your body when messages get scrambled? Nothing great. You may experience tremors, muscle weakness, stiffness, and spasms. You could have trouble with coordination, and fatigue may wear you down. It is not a simple or pleasant thing to realize that you cannot walk properly.

When nothing seems to balance, the best thing you can do is try to find the root cause of your balance problems. Is it your vision? Your ears? Your legs? Are you having a full on relapse? Then again, it could be a reaction to bad medication or a simple ear infection.

Involuntary Movements and Spasticity

One of the worst symptoms that you can pick up is when your muscles move involuntarily. These movements can range from twitching to severe spasticity.

These involuntary movements are called "dyskinesias," and there are quite a few types of them. With MS patients, sometimes the spasticity can be so bad that they end up tying themselves into knots.

- Athetosis is the writhing movement of your fingers and hands.
- Chorea are continuous jerky movements that linger for a few seconds after extension. They happen most often in limbs, the head, and the face.
- Dystonias are sustained muscle contractions that cause repetitive twisting movements and abnormal postures.
- Hemiballism are wild throwing movements with one arm or leg.
- Myoclonus are rapid muscle jerks that are frequently repetitive.
- Tremors are rhythmic movements of a part of your body. The

most common are kinetic or action tremors that occur when interacting with things. As your goal-directed hand moves toward an object, the tremor will worsen.

With MS spasticity and muscle spasms, you will feel stiffness in your arms and legs. It will make it difficult for you to move around. Spasticity occurs when muscle mass increases, and it happens mostly as night.

The intensity of your spasticity depends on your state of mind—like your stress level, posture, and position. Avoid wearing tight clothing, and avoid humidity and infections to control spasticity. Physical therapy and medication can be used; although if it happens often, you should treat it naturally by using stretching techniques.

Visual Disturbances and Speech Disruption

With Multiple Sclerosis, you could end up having some visual disturbances and speech problems during your lifetime. The key is to know how to handle them and to have a plan in place for when they happen.

People with MS may suffer with optic neuritis, double vision, and uncontrolled eye movements. For me, some days my vision was not clear. My optic nerve exam appeared to be normal; however, a CAT scan of the nerve of my right eye showed that I had changes. I still monitor these changes on a yearly basis and recommend you do the same with your ophthalmologist.

Speech problems are another symptom of MS. The brainstem is usually responsible for these issues. Scanning speech is when the normal rhythm or melody of speech is disrupted, causing elongated syllables and long words.

Slurring is another type of speech disturbance that may affect you. It is due to the muscle issues inherent in MS mouth, cheek, tongue, and lip movements. Nasal speech occurs when it sounds as though you are talking with a blocked nose but there is no blockage.

You can work on these speech problems with a language

pathologist, or you can take up a hobby learning to be a great orator for practice.

Pain Explored

Pain is hands down the worst symptom of MS, and it manifests in a host of different ways. Almost half of all multiple sclerosis patients suffer with chronic pain. As you know, this can lead to painkiller abuse and serious liver and kidney damage if left unchecked.

- Aching, tightness, or burning indicates neurologic pain in MS sufferers. While there are medications that can stop the pain, wearing stockings or pressure gloves can help. What works best is the use of plant-based anti-inflammatories, such as turmeric.

- Trigeminal neuralgia or stabbing pain in your face could be an initial symptom of MS. It can be alarming, but is easily treated with plant-based anti-inflammatories.

- Lhermitte's sign is a stabbing pain that runs along the back of your neck down your spine when you bend your neck forward. It feels like a shock of electricity coursing through you. I experienced Lhermitte's prior to my stumbling as one of the first signs on MS. Fortunately, Lhermitte's slowly fazes out.

Other pain like pins and needles and spasticity will always benefit from over-the-counter anti-inflammatory medications. However, natural, plant-based remedies are better to use since over-the-counter meds can cause liver and kidney complications. In addition, a daily stretching program is key in keeping muscles loose and decreasing spasticity. Aquatic therapy in a pool offers great benefits in rehabilitation.

Bladder and Bowel Dysfunction

One of the most common MS symptoms is constipation. It is best to deal with this by eating a high-fiber diet, drinking lots of water, and using mild stool softeners.

Multiple sclerosis patients are also known to develop bladder trouble, the least fashionable type of problem to deal with. This can manifest as a frequent and urgent need to urinate, problems beginning urination, incontinence, and frequent night time urination. It is best to avoid urinary tract infections by drinking lots of water—the amount in ounces equaling your weight divided by two.

Long-term problems like sleep disturbances and work-related embarrassment must be dealt with and planned for. Learning about bladder management is key to eliminating the probability that you will have kidney damage or infections through your life.

With MS come a lot of digestive concerns because your central nervous system does not deliver the right electrical impulses to the muscles that are charged with emptying your bowel. As a result, constipation is a constant battle.

Things like diet, not enough fiber, lack of physical activity, and tons of medication can make digestive concerns even worse for you. Some sufferers even develop bowel incontinence, which means that they do not get to the bathroom in time.

Diarrhea can cause a lot of issues if you are already having bladder and bowel trouble. Whatever you do, never cut back on your water intake as it will make things worse. With the right diet and exercise, you can get a handle on your bowel concerns.

Sexual Dysfunction

Unfortunately, MS also affects your sex drive because arousal begins in the central nervous system. If these pathways are damaged, you are going to have trouble becoming aroused and eventually reaching orgasm.

Men can experience issues maintaining erections, while women may experience reduced vaginal sensations, pain, or extreme dryness. This kind of sexual dysfunction is why many MS patients feel isolated from their partners after diagnosis.

And with 63% of people saying their sex drive dropped[19] after diagnosis, you are going to have to work extra hard to keep your partner happy. Otherwise, you may decide to use aids, like Viagra, or other specialist sexual arousal equipment.

Cognitive Disruption and Depression

I am very lucky that I have not suffered from cognitive disruption, but I have met many who have said their lives have been changed because of MS cognitive impairment.

Cognitive disruption is when your higher level brain functions are affected. This means that you will become more likely to forget things and unable to learn new things, understand and use language, shift attention, and perform calculations.

Everything from word finding, visual perception changes, memory, and executive functions will be tied into your MS diagnosis. You may experience one or two areas where you have the most trouble, or you could experience all areas.

The only way to prevent this is to dedicate yourself right now to consistent learning. Start reading and doing memory tests online. You can also enlist the help of a trained professional that will help you retain your language skills.

Depression is something that impacts some MS patients. Depression is an issue you can successfully manage and eliminate using psychiatric intervention and nutrition. Additionally, it is important to remember that exercise helps combat depression, as does playing games. I love to play cognitive games on Lumosity.com and enjoy the thrill of improving my score each week.

---

19   MS and Sex, http://msmeans.wordpress.com/sex-and-ms/

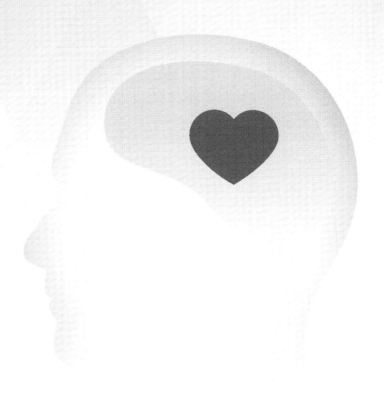

CHAPTER 4

Conventional Treatment, Extraordinary Pain

"Risk more than others think safe. Dream more than others think practical. Expect more than others think possible. Care more than others think wise."

HOWARD SHULTZ,
CHAIRMAN AND CEO OF STARBUCKS

We live in a world of conventional treatment, where doctors dish out prescribed, standard treatment options for diseases that have no cure and little evidence of recovery. Day after day, people are diagnosed with MS.

For the doctor, this is just another element of their day. For the patient, it begins a whirlwind journey of either recovery or degeneration. What happens to you is ultimately up to you, not your doctor. This chapter will tell you why that is the case.

That Moment You Are Diagnosed

I will never forget the moment I was diagnosed and how it impacted my life. With my husband at home and getting on in years—and me being diagnosed with MS at 60—I knew that the road ahead was going to be long and arduous.

In conventional medicine, when you are diagnosed, you are called into the doctor's office and sat down. The news is usually delivered in a quiet, even tone so that you do not get too upset by it. The doctors will walk you through what the tests found and why he or she believes that you have multiple sclerosis.

What the Doctor Likes to Tell You

As a doctor and someone who has been diagnosed with MS, I have a unique perspective on both sides of the diagnosis process. It can be very stressful for doctors to have to deliver such terrible news to patients, and it often happens at times of great trouble.

It is uncommon that people with an MS diagnosis are "fine." Often it is emergency room visits, severe physical trauma, or some other issue that has forced them to try to find an answer. When it comes, doctors can unwittingly make the situation worse.

For a host of reasons, doctors will often downplay your symptoms or diagnosis. Whether it is because of their own mental state, comparisons they are making between you and other patients, or perhaps the need to deliver harsh news in a kind way, it confuses the patient.

These circumstances are not unique; reports are published[20] on the way doctors deal with patient symptoms and diagnosis all the time. But it leads patients to the wrong conclusions about their illness and can set them on the wrong path.

Once you have been diagnosed, your doctor will recommend that you immediately begin taking injections of a drug to help "stabilize" your MS. I was on these injections for some time, and I can tell you that they did not help. In fact, they made me worse in many ways.

Doctors are wonderful people, but they have to deal with the business side of medicine—which means prescribing drugs that they endorse and keeping the pharmaceutical companies and reps happy. You could end up on a drug that does more harm than good.

---

20   Denise Grady, In Reporting Symptoms, Don't Patients Know Best?, http://www.nytimes.com/2010/04/13/health/13seco.html?ref=health

When I experienced the lack of progress with drug therapy for myself, I decided to try my own alternative treatments. The more I read about alternative treatment, the more viable it sounded. I wanted to explore, to reeducate myself, and to inspire myself to find solutions where there were none. On this journey, I learned so much about food, dense nutrients, and genetically modified soy.

The bottom line was that drug treatments came with a long list of complications, while nutritional adjustments came with none. After trying the modern medicine route, I knew the only way to find the truth would be to put effort into alternative treatment.

Reductionist Medicine: A Modern Inconvenience?

Anyone with an MS diagnosis will tell you that the symptoms are so varied and strange that it can feel like your whole body is under attack sometimes. And therein lies the problem when you choose to listen to your doctor and take their prescribed treatments.

The current Western medical system is built on reductionist[21] principles, which means that doctors are taught to look at "pieces of a system" instead of the whole system. This is why you had to go to see so many specialists before you could get diagnosed.

There are doctors for every part of you, and they all practice their special branch of medicine—while largely ignoring the rest. The human body, I have discovered, does not align with this type of medical reasoning as well as I might have hoped.

While reductionist medicine has done a ton of good for many diseases, it has also led to the "drug and dice" culture. If you journey across the sea to Asia, the treatments there are more holistic, meaning that they look at your whole body when trying to fix an issue.

---

21   Holism vs. Reductionism: Comparing the Fundamentals of Conventional and Alternative Medicinal Modalities, http://exploreim.ucla.edu/education/holism-vs-reductionism-comparing-the-fundamentals-of-conventional-and-alternative-medicinal-modalities/

For patients with MS, reductionist medicine can be a modern black hole. It is the reason why you had to endure so many tests and so many hospital visits. Because MS attacks the nerves, putting unhealthy drugs and treatments in your body can and does aggravate your situation. You can end up feeling worse and getting worse if you are not careful.

It is unfortunate that you as the patient are subject to the biases of your doctor or care provider. The important thing is that you understand that your doctor is a human being and they make mistakes. They do not know your body like you do, and they do not experience the side effects of their decisions.

Surviving in an Age of Non Self-Responsibility

In Western culture, trusting your doctor is as normal as trusting a teacher—only with much greater consequences. Doctors have always had an authority about them that makes people respect and care about their direction and opinions.

As a doctor, I have experienced this many times. People will take your advice, and they will take it as the "only method" of treatment because it came from you, someone they trust. But as I discovered, there is more to this relationship than doctors see.

We are living in an age of non-responsibility, where people believe that if their doctors cannot fix them, they cannot be fixed. People have become so afraid of venturing out and trying to treat themselves on their own.

When you look around and see the whole picture, it is a scary thing. Ill health is rampant, and all that these "sick" people care about is visiting the doctor to get drugs or procedures that will make them "well" again. They do not want to deal with the consequences of their own lifestyle choices.

For an MS sufferer, if you are going to survive in this age of blatant non-responsibility, you need to look at yourself. How have you lived to cause these effects in your body? Perhaps the disease can be controlled if only you look for solutions outside of your doctor.

Thankfully, many people are doing just that. It is the reason why you chose to buy this book and make a change. You need to realize, like I did, that *you* are responsible for your own health and wellness. You need to make positive changes to correct this deficit, or your doctor will do their best—and there is every chance that you will suffer for it.

The Elephant in the Room: Knowing Your Options

Like so many doctors before me, I dismissed the benefits of alternative medicine. Being a doctor, I was sure that I would be able to find a treatment or a cure for myself in the world of medicine, but boy, was I mistaken.

My wish is that MS patients like you have the courage to explore all of your options after you are diagnosed. Simply listening to what your doctors says and loading your body with drugs is not going to make anything better.

It is up to you to understand what it is they are prescribing and how it will affect your body. It is important to weigh the negative and positive elements of the medication before you take it. Sometimes the risks far outweigh any benefits, especially when you hear the stats on how the medicine works. Success rates are few.

The elephant in the room is always going to be the fact that doctors adhere to conventional medicine and side line alternative medicine. They would rather drug you or send you for surgery than help you explore alternative methods of getting better.

The real tragedy is that these doctors have no real idea how much of a positive impact that alterative healing can have for a patient with MS. The success and improvement rates for these treatments may not be widespread yet, but I have never spoken to an MS sufferer that did not benefit from knowing all of their treatment possibilities.

The truth is that many side effects of conventional treatments may threaten your life and can make your MS worse. Everyone is different, but for every person that benefits briefly from treatment, there is a person in pain from a side effect. Compare that to alternative medicine, which has almost no side effects.

The Unclear Causes of MS

No one knows what causes MS. It is not due to lack of study but rather the complex nature of the disease and how it differs from person to person. Some people go through their whole lives with MS, and no real symptoms manifest.

Others can barely walk, or see, by 30. It really depends on several critical factors that science has determined thus far. For example:

- *Immune system factors* – When your central nervous system attacks the myelin coating around your nerves (and your nerves themselves), it is known as an abnormal immune mediated response. Scientists are investigating why some T cells are attracted to myelin, what causes it, and how it can be slowed or stopped.

- *Genetic factors* – Like many other diseases, if a parent or sibling has MS, the chances of you developing it later on are that much higher. Some genes are triggered by environmental factors to cause MS, and this is being studied at great length by scientists.

- *Environmental factors* – A number of factors are taken into account here, including age, gender, ethnic background, proximity to the equator, demographics, geography, genetics, and infectious causes. Smoking and not getting enough vitamin D are two causes that are being thoroughly investigated.

- *Infectious factors* – Lots of bacteria and viruses have been researched to play a role in the later development of MS. Epstein-Barr virus (glandular fever), measles, human herpes, and chlamydia have all been known to precede diagnosis.

Your doctor probably told you that there are no certain causes of MS. Your environment, your injury and illness history, and your genetics will all have played a part in it. Studies have shown, however, that one of the reasons why women get it more than men is because of their sex hormones.

Higher level of estrogen and progesterone can suppress your immune system function. It also may explain why during pregnancy, MS sufferers have barely any symptoms.

Multiple sclerosis is different for everyone, which is why early symptoms are often misdiagnosed or impossible to detect. The signs, however, are there. Multiple visits to the doctor, uncertainty, lots of tests—nearly all MS patients go through this. Below are the most common early signs of MS, which could or could not display themselves at the same time.

- *Problems with your vision.* MS causes optic neuritis, which is inflammation of your optic nerve. It causes blurred vision, particularly in one eye.
- *Numb, tingling sensations on your body.* If you feel strange sensations like tingling, burning, crawling, or loss of sensation, it could be MS. Resistance or intense response to heat and cold are also common.
- *Muscle weakness and spasms.* If your limbs feel heavy and clumsy, it could be a sign of MS. Some 40% of all MS patients begin with spasms and stiffness in their legs.
- *Fatigue is common.* One of the worst symptoms of MS is fatigue. If you are exhausted by the early afternoon, it may be MS. Even though this only happens in about 20% of MS patients,[22] nearly all MS sufferers develop it at some point.
- *Balance and coordination problems.* Difficulty walking normally and maintaining their balance is a sign of early onset

---

22   Multiple Sclerosis In-Depth Report, http://www.nytimes.com/health/guides/disease/multiple-sclerosis/print.html

MS. Tremors and having trouble grasping objects is also a common occurrence.

Other symptoms may develop, including shooting, stabbing, or intermittent pain and speech problems. Mood swings, cognitive issues, and digestive system concerns are also precursors to the disease. You may have had one or all of these symptoms before you were diagnosed.

Why Doctors Dismiss Natural Medicine

Since the 1920s the American Medical Association has tried extremely hard to shut down the naturopathic, alternative, and chiropractic branches of medicine in the U.S.[23] Anyone that has brought up natural treatments with their doctor realizes that the response they get is often hostile or ends up in the doctor making the patient feel "silly" for bringing it up.

There are very good reasons why doctors dislike natural medicine so much. This does not mean that these alternative medicine sources are bad; quite the opposite. The source of much of this conflict revolves around money. Doctors belong to medical groups, hospitals, and associations, and when people start healing themselves, they lose income.

This has been well documented with the plummeting numbers of general practitioners[24] in America. They have been the first to feel the "holistic health boom," and because of that, young doctors are choosing to study specializations instead.

23   Erika Janik, The Battle for Medicine's Soul: A Century of Alternative Remedies, http://www.salon.com/2014/01/19/the_battle_for_medicines_soul_a_century_of_alternative_remedies/

24   Marina Koren, America Is Running Out of Doctors, http://www.nationaljournal.com/health-care/america-is-running-out-of-doctors-20131104

A fascinating look at how doctors treat themselves, as opposed to patients, is quite revealing. Many studies[25] have been conducted proving that doctors almost never take their own advice. When faced with the same scenario, they often cast off the invasive procedures and drugs—and instead opt for natural medicine themselves!

Natural medicine reduces their income, endangers their jobs, and places the patient's life at risk. Most doctors will insist that you at least try a treatment, but do not be bullied into anything until you have seen the success rates. They will astound you.

MS From the Perspective of a Doctor-Patient

Doctors, alternative healers—everyone will agree that MS is not like other diseases. It affects your whole body and can be triggered by the smallest of things. Your lifestyle and what you put into your body becomes of paramount importance when this is the case.

As a doctor-patient, I can tell you that I experienced more relief, greater health, and much improved stamina after doing my own investigations into natural treatments. These natural treatments did far more for me than *any* of the drugs or procedures my doctor put me on or suggested. I am still astounded that these treatments are not offered to patients.

Multiple sclerosis cannot be cured, but it can be reduced to the point where you do not even realize that it is there anymore. You can manage your MS to the point where your quality of life drastically improves over time. It all begins with alternative treatment.

As a doctor, the last thing I was expecting to find was such a simple, affordable, and effective route to managing such a serious illness. But I have made enquiries and realize that almost everyone else that commits to management through alternative means gets the help they need. This is incredible when you consider that some MS

---

25   Elizabeth Renter, "Mainstream" Doctors and Nurses Often Use Alternative Medicine for Themselves, http://naturalsociety.com/doctors-and-nurses-often-prefer-alternative-medicine/

patients are bedridden.

The "us vs. them" conflict that rages on between the conventional medicine camp and the alternative medicine camp becomes your fight when you are diagnosed. The key is to discover the treatments that will help you and make your body stronger over time.

One thing I understand now is that even the smallest pill can have a long-term consequence. Try to see your body as completely unique. You are not cattle, and there is no such thing as a "cure all." All you can do is test what works and use it.

The Problems with Modern Treatments

There are a lot of issues with modern treatments that MS patients do not understand. This can lead you to embrace a new drug or procedure that does not help you recover or improve your MS. It is so important to understand what you are doing to your body.

The first issue is that your doctor or the hospital that you are at may insist on putting you on a course of these medications. Sometimes patients can become physically dependent on them, or they may cause you to need stronger and stronger medicine down the line.

With each new "pill" or "injection" or "procedure" that comes out, you will hear how it changed people's lives and fixed their MS. This is because the giant marketing machine that promotes these treatments wants you to buy them.

More and more online, it has become difficult to find real information about MS treatments because pharmaceutical companies are using their considerable marketing might to secure top spots on all of the search engines. They literally drown out the negative feedback that patients want others to know about.

Most MS drugs have strengths and weaknesses. Several years ago, there were only nine main drugs on the market, and they had horrific side effects. These days there are more drugs available—with fewer side effects—but you should be no less suspicious of them.

I have yet to find any drugs at all that compare with the results that a patient can get from streamlining their diet, exercising regularly, and controlling their stress levels. And that is ultimately the problem. Until a modern treatment can out-perform natural treatments, there is no real reason to flood your body with those side effects.

The Roadblocks to Natural Healing

When a patient says to their doctor that they are going to try "alternative" treatments and natural healing, the doctor will almost always shake their head in disbelief. This is because most doctors do not believe that the average person has the discipline required to effect any positive change on their own bodies.

There are some serious roadblocks to healing yourself naturally, as you will discover. The first and the most important is self-responsibility. You cannot treat your new food and exercise regimen lightly; it is the medicine that you are giving your body to heal.

That means cutting out all forms of sugar, junk food, and processed food that could trigger a relapse. It means understanding that your *choices* are crucial in your healing process. You need to upgrade your lifestyle if you are going to have any shot at getting better.

Being a doctor, I was used to strict training and regimens. You might find the process a struggle, but if you want the results, you must stick to the plan. Roadblocks include eating the wrong things, not exercising enough, not looking after yourself, not resting, and not managing your stress levels. These are critical to your recovery process. That means choosing the right food, the right exercises, and the right techniques for relaxation and finding the best supplements to enhance your physical health. There are many other societal roadblocks you will have to face, too.

I struggled on the raw food diet, but I was lucky in that I am naturally a very disciplined person, so I could make it work. Many other people may find it a long, hard road. You have to evaluate the pros and cons and take the time to understand what will happen to you if you do not. Quality of life means testing different things when there are no clear answers.

It is scary finding your own treatments, and people will urge you to follow your doctor's advice and treatment plan. Your doctor may not be happy with you, and you might have to go through some hard lessons to figure out what works and what does not. But all of this still does less damage than traditional treatments.

When Alternative Is All You Have Left: Positive Change

Not only am I a doctor but I also went through the process of being on the doctor-recommended drugs. I was afraid, and the only comfort was my doctor, who had a plan. So I did what most people do, and I followed it for a while.

The drug therapies did nothing for me. I did not improve, but my overall health was significantly degenerating. The results that I got back from the drugs are not even worth mentioning other than the horrible lipdystrophy side effects that persist to this day.

I looked into other treatments like CCSVI, or chronic cerebrospinal venous insufficiency, which an Italian doctor suggested may be the cause of MS. When there is an abnormality in blood drainage from the brain to the spinal cord, it could cause the nerve damage in MS.

I also did a ton of research on stem cell treatments, but this new science is still being studied and is getting off the ground. I reached the point where I had investigated everything, tried everything I could, and still nothing worked.

Being a doctor, I knew that things would not get better if I did not take action. So I was forced to investigate natural treatments for MS. Alternative medicine was literally all I had left. I am so glad now that I decided to turn to natural therapies, as they have raised my quality of life and saved me from living with degenerating MS.

I know in my heart that they can do the same thing for you. This is positive change in the purest sense—medicine that does not harm but heals your body on so many levels. As you continue to read this book, think about embracing alternative healing to treat your MS or—at the very least—test it for a few months.

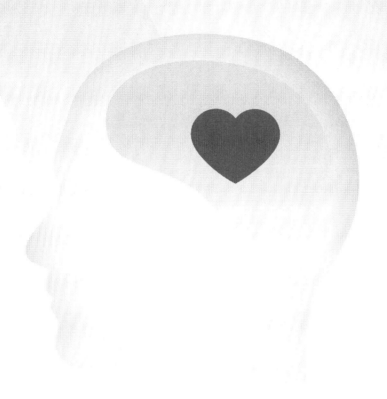

CHAPTER **5**

Turning Point: A Mind for Curious Investigations

"Opportunity is missed by people because it is dressed in overalls and looks like work."

THOMAS EDISON

The moment you are diagnosed all that matters is finding the cure. As far as I know, there is no cure that exists right now. But there is something almost as good as the cure, and that is having a mind for curious investigations.

People with MS that stay up to date on the latest treatments, both natural and conventional, are positioned to benefit first if a cure is ever discovered. And sometimes, the right treatment can be just as good as a cure.

Keeping an Ear to the Ground: Cure?

So far modern science has developed a host of drug treatments and invasive procedures to slow the progression of MS, minimize the symptoms, and improve physical and mental function. In other words, to help you manage your MS for quality of life.

While there is no cure, there are several treatments that are moving forward and may be beneficial in the future. Some of these are:

- *Teriflunomide:* A disease-modifier under the brand "Aubagio" has been approved for use in the U.S. The *New England Journal of Medicine* found that people that took this drug showed significantly lower disease progression than the control group, which was taking placebos.

- *Dimethyl Fumarate:* Another disease modifier under the brand "Tecfidera" stops your immune system from attacking itself and destroying your myelin. It also has a protective effect on the body.

- *Dalfampridine:* This blocks the potassium channels in your nerves to improve conductivity. The drug is said to improve walking speed, but the studies are unclear.

- *Modified Story Technique:* To restore cognitive function, the Kessler Foundation Research Center developed a technique to rehabilitate people suffering from the cognitive effects of MS.

Nervous System Damage: CCSVI

CCSVI, or chronic cerebrospinal venous insufficiency, is a condition that one doctor linked to MS as the potential cause. Dr. Paolo Zamboni, an Italian doctor, conducted a study that suggested all MS patients have irregular neck veins.

Blood flow from the brain to the central nervous system is compromised, which causes iron deposits around the pulmonary veins. This in turn triggers the autoimmunity and the eventual degeneration of myelin.

While this study was fascinating and interesting, it did have some methodological issues. The test group was too small, and the study was not random or blinded. The participants remained on their normal treatment plans during the test.

This muddied the cause and effect of the study—and all of the subjects were in the relapse phase—which meant that a recovery was going to happen anyway. Dr. Zamboni[26] cleared away the blockages using angioplasty, with most subjects improving some six months after the procedure was done.

Unfortunately, at 18 months many participants were doing worse than they had before, with some having no change at all. This story relates back to the original problems with reductionist medicine and using doctor treatments—money.

As it turns out, Dr. Zamboni owns a patent for the diagnostic equipment used for diagnosing CCSVI. But this does not completely invalidate his research, which is why the many MS foundations are supporting his work and funding additional studies.

I went in for CCSVI after researching it extensively. I booked myself into the Hubbard Foundation in San Diego, California, although at the time, I was living in Panama. I had read a lot about CCSVI and believed that it had some merit. At the time, I had tremendous urinary incontinence, so the risk was worth it.

I scheduled an appointment for this experimental procedure and had it done. It was not traumatic, and it was quick. I had a local anesthetic followed by a functional MRI to show the before and after shots. The whole thing took about an hour. The facility was nice, I was monitored the entire time, and it turns out that one of my jugular veins was obstructed. This prevented blood from flowing correctly to my brain.

Interestingly, it did improve my MS (especially urinary incontinence) for the first month by about 80%, then it slowly undid itself. At the end of that month, I was back to where I had been. Later, I attended a lecture on MS and was told that 60% of MS patients are placebo responders, which I could have been after the treatment. I went back and had another MRI.

As suspected, the vein had reocculded, which had brought my

---

26   Paulo Zamboni, The Big Idea: Iron-Dependent Inflammation in Venous Disease and Proposed Parallels in Multiple Sclerosis, http://jrs.sagepub.com/content/99/11/589.long

symptoms back. I could have had it done again, but the first three thousand dollars seemed enough. The science and evidence just was not there. A friend of mine had it done too, with little impact. It was time to move on.

Officially, CCSVI treatment is being studied. Do not rush out to get it, as people have died from complications.[27] The best thing is to wait and see what the medical community finds out about this procedure or to wait for an NIH trial.

Reaching Out: Stem Cell Adventures

A much more likely cure points to stem cells. I have researched them heavily and am very interested in the stem cells trials that are going on all over the globe. Stem cells are cells that can both reproduce themselves and eventually become any other kind of cell.

The potential to use stem cells to treat MS is very real. The only stumbling block is that these tests are still being conducted and studies are on the go. The researchers that are actively involved in these trials believe that stem cells can be used to fix two core issues.

The first is to repair or completely replace the damaged tissue in your body. The brain and spinal cord will be repaired by re-growing the myelin so that your nerve fibers are once again protected from damage.

The second is to replace your immune system, which does not work properly in patients with MS. By doing this, the patient will not experience any more damage. Together, the two combine to be a complete cure for multiple sclerosis.

Unfortunately, even though the studies are indicating good things, so far only people involved in clinical trials can benefit from these treatments. It is not available to the broad public, and when it does eventually become available, it will probably cost a sizable amount.

---

27   Deena Beasley, Genevra Pittman, FDA Cites Risk, but MS Patients Seek Unproven Therapy, http://www.reuters.com/article/2012/10/05/us-usa-health-ms-idUSBRE89416320121005

The most recent study will determine how safe the treatment is for widespread use and how effective the treatments are. Preclinical testing showed[28] that after injecting the stem cells, brain inflammation was reduced in seven MS patients, myelin was repaired, and protection of the neuronal structure and function of the brain was improved.

I visited a stem cell institute in Panama to find out more, as procedures in the U.S. are restricted. There is a future in stem cells, but they still need to be studied and well documented. The stem cells come from the umbilical cord of a healthy infant, but because the circumstances had to be just right, I chose not to do it for myself. The transplant is expensive, and I could not make sense of the promise that these cells would regrow my myelin, so I will wait for improved research in the future.

The Research on Natural MS Treatments

One of the most profound things I ever realized was that the human body wants to heal itself. You have everything you need to heal as long as you are putting in the work. The "work" is all about the right nutrition, proper supplementation, exercise, stress management, and meditation.

MS is a variable disease, with no two people experiencing the same symptoms. There is progressive MS, and exacerbation and remission MS, and a type of MS that does not produce any major symptoms at all.

Because of the disease's variability, patients respond well to natural treatments. These can include any number of healing practices.

- Remove milk and milk products from your diet.
- Eat locally grown vegetables and fruits.
- Eat very little meat, preferably grass-fed.

---

28 Groundbreaking Multiple Sclerosis Stem Cell Trial Approved, http://www.medicalnewstoday.com/articles/264892.php

- Only consume organically grown, non-hormone, non-antibiotic foods.
- Cut out sugar, wheat, and gluten.
- Remove all processed food from your diet.
- Take supplements such as antioxidants, B vitamins, Omega 3, vitamin C, and CoQ 10.
- Do exercises such as yoga, stretching, aquatic therapy, or light weights.[29]

Experiment with yoga and Pilates; these are slow, measured exercises that improve your health and strengthen your body. Many MS patients say that when they stop doing yoga, they have a relapse. Practice de-stressing techniques like visualization, meditation, and hypnotherapy, and investigate Eastern medicine.

Yoga reduces fatigue in MS patients, according to a study from the Oregon Health & Science University study.[30] Practicing yoga every day is ideal for reducing your stress levels, increasing blood flow, and improving your health with MS.

More of That Healing Research

A major study was conducted by the University of Copenhagen that mapped out how natural treatments can help manage MS. This study included things like acupuncture, herbal treatments, and dietary supplements. The study showed that people tend to use these treatments as strengthening and preventative measures.

Acupuncture, the practice of placing needles into the human body at strategic points, has been proven to help patients with MS. Fatigue in particular is remedied, as proven in many studies.[31]

29   Randomized Controlled Trial of Yoga and Exercise in Multiple Sclerosis, http://www.uvm.edu/~rsingle/JournalClub/papers/Oken%2BNeurology-2004_MS%2Byoga.pdf

30   Yoga Reduces Fatigue in MS Patients, OHSU Study Finds, http://www.ohsu.edu/xd/about/news_events/news/2004/06-08-yoga-reduces-fatigue-in.cfm

31   Amantadine and the Place of Acupuncture in the Treatment of Fatigue in Patients With

Ayurvedic medicine translates to mean "the science of life" and can be a particularly restorative form of treatment for MS patients. This is because the many dietary and lifestyle changes positively affect the human body. Ayurvedic medicine also harnesses yoga, meditation, massage, exercise, and balancing nutrition to heal.

Some studies have been conducted on different elements within Ayurvedic medicine,[32] and they have found that it can be helpful in treating pain, anxiety, depression, spasticity, and fatigue. Be careful to avoid some practitioners and remedies that often have heavy metals in them. Make sure that your practitioner is qualified.

There are dozens of nutritional studies that support the notion that controlling your diet leads to MS recovery. Particular studies to note are Professor Roy Laver Swank's work[33] on dietary fats and how MS patients should not drink milk or eat saturated fat of any kind.

Natural supplements have been found by many studies to improve quality of life for MS patients. A study in Cyprus concluded that there is a 64% reduction in relapse risk when taking a combination of supplements. These included Omega 3, antioxidants, B 12, and vitamin E. I highly recommend finding a supplement cocktail that works for you.

Comparing Modern Treatments with Natural Treatments

That means if you go off the medication, you may have secondary concerns to deal with. Right now, if MS is your only concern, begin with the natural healing process. If it does not work for you or you lose faith in it, you can always switch to modern medicine.

On the other side of the spectrum, these modern treatments are relatively quick. The trade-off is to substitute them for natural

---

Multiple Sclerosis: An Observational Study, http://www.ncbi.nlm.nih.gov/pubmed/23151355

32   Ayurveda, http://www.neurologycare.net/ayurveda.html

33   Diet, http://www.overcomingmultiplesclerosis.org/Recovery-Program/Diet

treatments that need time every day, that must be followed in a disciplined manner, and that have almost no side effects.

In fact, the only side effects that you get from things like dietary supplements, proper nutrition, and exercise are all beneficial. Your body will grow in strength, and your stress levels will rapidly decline. This is great news for MS patients.

So I would be hesitant to compare the two, just as I would be hesitant to try only one. Everybody is different, and you may seriously need modern medication. But I urge you to test the natural healing theory first as a control. Otherwise you will never know how bad it really gets when you start taking that medication.

Hopefully, in the future, both types of medicine become one, and the patient is once again placed at the center of the treatment.

A World of Possibility: Simple Works

During my long testing process trying out different techniques, medications, and natural treatments, I discovered that as long as I was keeping my body healthy, my MS was under control. This is a very important fact that doctors do not like to talk about.

There is a world of possibility out there right now, where you can find amazing natural treatments that calm, restore, and treat your MS. They may sound simple, but there is a very good reason why they have been used to treat illness for hundreds of years.

The world is full of plants and herbs; you only need to create your own test environments to see if they work for you. To do this, make sure that you are not on any medication or other treatments at the time.

Record what you take or what you do and how you feel every day for three months. This will give your body enough time to adjust. The good news is that most herbs will not cause any negative side effects if you take them in recommended doses.

There may be treatments that I have not heard of that you discover.

If this happens, make sure that you put in the time to find out if these treatments are feasible, and then do a trial test run. After a year, you will know exactly what works best with your MS and your body.

Most of all, look for who funds these studies, and try to get to the root cause of why a particular person or group is advocating for a specific product. Often you will find that you take an herb that does nothing but has a great reputation. That is just marketing, so move on.

The Healing Power of Alternative Health

When you want to find the root cause of your ill health, you do not have to look any further than the food you eat, the environment you live in, and the products you use. It is no coincidence that there is more disease now than ever before.

There are many incredible treatments that you can try that will rapidly improve your health and wellness. I know because I have tried them, and they work.

More than that, these treatments work better than any medication I ever took. That may just be because of my physiology, but I believe it runs much deeper than that. Using a drug that barely works and makes you sicker over time is no long-term healing strategy.

But it makes sense to infuse your body with health and treat it like it is supposed to be treated. Taking alternative medicines and performing age-old practices realigns you with what is important. There is healing power in a combination of these factors.

Just making sure that your vitamin D levels are all right is instrumental in maintaining good health. Most people with MS have low vitamin D levels, which is actually a precursor to the disease. If a doctor had caught your low vitamin D levels, you may have been able to fix them. Repairing this deficiency instantly improves your vitality.

Doctors will not screen for these things, so you will have to go to a certified natural health specialist, who will run a host of blood tests to see how your body is using nutrition and how you can fix all of those little problems. There is real power in that.

Couple it with exercise and relaxation, and you are looking at a natural, side effect-free way to manage your MS. I only wish someone had told me this before I took the medication.

What MS Researchers Are Working On

It is important for you to stay abreast of the current trends in the medical world of MS research and discovery. New drugs are being launched all the time, and new treatments are being created for testing.

Here is some of the latest research that I have uncovered for you.

- Low Dose Naltrexone, or LDN, has been found to trigger a prolonged up-regulation of endorphins. This has an anti-inflammatory effect that can help treat and ease the symptoms of MS. Small clinical trials are positive, showing a significant reduction in spasticity for patients.
- Vitamin D deficiency is being studied as a cause of MS. This is because most MS patients live away from the equator and tend to be in cold climates. If you wear sunscreen, consider taking a vitamin D supplement.
- Oral cannabinoids from medical cannabis is being studied to see if it relieves most of the major symptoms of MS.

Researchers all over the world are conducting studies on how to cure MS and manage it as well as how to prevent kids from developing MS in later life. Keeping an eye on the latest research will help you make important decisions throughout your life.

Waiting for the Cure: A Life on Hold

Sometimes it seems as though modern science is moments away from a cure. Other times hope feels like wasted energy. I guess it depends on the progression of your disease and how well you are able to cope with it.

The hard truth is that many drug companies compete for a place in the market. Even if a drug is profoundly successful, red tape may keep it from hitting the market for 30 years.[34] There is no guarantee that a cure will come in your lifetime.

The best that you can do is change your life right now so that your body can heal itself and fight against the disease. This is something everyone can do, and while it is not easy at times, the physical benefits are long lasting and wonderful.

The worst thing that you can do is nothing because many types of MS end up in paralysis and severe disability. You have to make a choice to heal yourself as well as you can while you can. If that means fighting against pain to do yoga, then do it!

Waiting for a cure is something millions of people around the world are familiar with. But no one really knows when it is going to happen or if it is ever going to happen. The best you can do is resign yourself to the fact that your body needs to focus on strength and health.

Putting your life on hold for MS may seem to be your only alternative. For many years, I was in denial about my disease process and did not seek any solutions. But once I found a path and remedies that worked for me, I achieved a better quality of life. You can do the same! If I can do it at 60, you can certainly do it, too.

The Reasons Why I Chose Life

When I was diagnosed, there was a long time when I felt that MS would get the better of me and I would end up disabled and unable to care for myself or my aging husband. It was actually my husband who motivated me to keep going.

---

34   Thirty-Year Wait for Multiple Sclerosis Drug Drags On, http://www.adelaidenow.com.au/news/south-australia/thirtyyear-wait-for-multiple-sclerosis-drug-drags-on/story-fni6uo1m-1226817956976

I had always been a workaholic, and stepping back from that was difficult. Even more difficult was the struggle to try to heal my MS. I was already experiencing symptoms of age, and when you have worked hard and long, it can be tough to separate them from your MS symptoms.

But I believe that all MS sufferers have a choice: traditional or alternative medicine. In so doing, we choose to be responsible for our quality of life. For me, it is important to be aware of the consequences of my choices, so I spent a lot of time studying the pros and cons of all of my options.

Choosing life is about seizing control of your disease. If I had not researched and implemented the natural health treatments in my own life, who knows how mobile I would be now. I know one thing for certain—and that is that MS can either rule you or motivate you!

Good nutrition and the right stress management techniques saved me. I had no idea that stress was causing that much of a physical consequence in my body. I believe that many people do not fully understand that until they work on solving the problem.

I encourage you to take this challenge and choose life, like I did. I am no different from anyone else, and my diagnosis does not define me. You can choose to do the same thing.

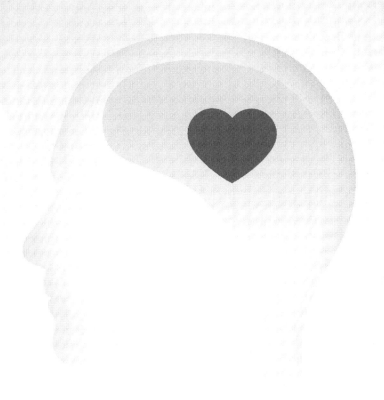

CHAPTER 6

The Path of Great Resistance: Being a Guinea Pig

"No matter what you're going through, there's a light at the end of the tunnel and it may seem hard to get to it but you can do it and just keep working towards it and you'll find the positive side of things."

DEMI LOVATO

There are many ways to treat multiple sclerosis, as you know, but first you need to come to terms with the idea that much of the time the treatments that you try will rely on how far you are willing to go to improve your health. That means becoming something of a guinea pig and going against conventional treatment options. But far from this being a scary journey, I have found that it is enlightening and inspiring, and it feeds the soul to take action against a disease that threatens your physical freedom.

Figuring Out the Nutrition Trap

It is true that MS is a degenerative disease. When you speak to your doctor about what your options are, they probably will not mention diet and exercise; no doctor mentioned either of these to me. I have found that there are certain foods that are best avoided and some that are best included in your diet more often.

It is also true that statistically speaking, no particular diet for MS has been proven[35] to be effective just yet. Malnutrition, however, can seriously exacerbate your multiple sclerosis symptoms! Nutrition in our modern society is not as it once was, and this becomes vital information for someone who could be lacking vitamins that could help your MS.

Back in 1970, vegetables were higher in nutrient value[36] than the vegetables being grown and harvested today. Even if you stop eating a poor diet of high saturated fat, high sugar, and high carbohydrate junk food and switch to natural, healthy foods, you may still encounter nutritional issues.

The truth is that Americans are getting fatter from junk food, and our health is rapidly declining. In the same breath, healthy Americans are still going without proper nutrition because food sources are not what they once were. For an individual like you with MS, nutrition is a lifeline that can reduce a host of symptoms that steal away your energy.

This is why I believe that there is a nutrition trap currently at play for people with MS. It is not enough to quit junk food and processed items; you also need to add a lot of new organic vegetables and fruit to your diet while carefully selecting high-quality proteins. Then you should also seriously consider a supplement routine to get enough vitamins into your diet.

What Doctors Don't Tell You About Nutrition

Nutrition is fast becoming the key to unlocking health in people with MS. But nutrition is something that is taking a back seat in medical institutions all over America out of budgetary need. The

---

35   Stefan Schwarz, Multiple Sclerosis and Nutrition, http://www.pinnaclife.com/sites/default/files/research/MS_and_Nutrition.pdf

36   Dirt Poor: Have Fruits and Vegetables Become Less Nutritious?, http://www.scientificamerican.com/article/soil-depletion-and-nutrition-loss/

hours devoted to educating doctors on nutrition are decreasing, which means that doctors are becoming ill-equipped to provide nutritional advice.[37]

This is absolutely not the doctor's fault, but it is causing limitations when MS patients have questions about a specific diet that could be helping them or could harm them. With so much new research emerging about the benefits of certain diets, questions have already been raised about why the medical establishment is not including this in their education system.

Nutrition, therefore, is something that doctors recommend as "lifestyle advice," but they do not consider it a viable treatment option. As far as they are concerned, you should already be eating healthy meals every day. Warnings are given, but little is done to express the real impact that nutrition can have for patients with MS.

When you combine the lack of education with the emerging research, it becomes clear that it is your responsibility as a patient with MS to find out what sort of nutrition you should be consuming or cutting out on a daily basis. When I found the right nutritional balance, it gave me my life back.

Personal experience, however, does little to persuade people when their doctors are offering them alternatives that have nothing to do with food. That is why I strongly suggest that you begin to see food as a method of treatment and not just something that you enjoy that will keep you moving and going.

MS patients will need coaching and support for nutritional matters in the future, but until the medical industry takes an active role, the onus is on you.

I have personally experienced the benefits of nutrition and the fact that what you put into your mouth affects your entire body. All

---

37   Julie Deardorff, Prescription for Nutrition, http://articles.chicagotribune.com/2013-03-26/health/ct-met-heart-nutrition-20130326_1_mediterranean-style-diet-heart-disease-diet-and-nutrition

levels are affected, especially your immune system. If your immune system does not work correctly, it affects your GI tracts and the basic metabolism of your body. Your insulin levels are impacted, and these control the entire regulatory system of blood sugar and hormones in the human body. Nutrition, in my opinion, is the single most important healing element to consider.

It does not surprise me that the level of auto immune diseases has escalated. Obesity and many of these other diseases are directly related to our food consumption. If you want to impact your health, change your perspective. American diets focus on carbs, sugar, wheat, and gluten—cut them out! If you are ill, the best advice I can give you is to focus on your food.

Figuring Out the Diet Trap

When someone tells you to diet, it conjures images of starvation, deprivation, and painfully long weeks of waning willpower. According to *Psychology Today*,[38] defined, it is known as "a temporary and highly restrictive program of eating in order to lose weight."

Think back to the days of the Atkins Diet, Weight Watchers, or Weigh Less—but the impression is always the use of food to lose fat. Interestingly, dieting in this context does not work. Almost all people that diet lose weight and then regain it within a period of five years.

When you have MS, your diet refers to the kinds of food that you choose, prepare, cook, and eat to maintain a balanced lifestyle and reduce your symptoms. Too often the old definition of dieting comes back into play, and it is not going to work for you like that.

The diet trap needs to be avoided. That means reframing the way you think about food and how your body uses it for health and wellness. It means dispelling your old belief that dieting is a short-term solution with an ending in the future.

---

38   Meg Selig, Why Diets Don't Work…and What Does, http://www.psychologytoday.com/blog/changepower/201010/why-diets-dont-workand-what-does

When you have MS, there is no such thing as eating a good diet for a while then going back to your usual junk food—not without serious symptom resurgences anyway. The trap here is that you will treat nutrition like it is a diet, and you will not be able to maintain that diet due to the restrictions and mindset that you have about dieting in general.

Diets that are too severe trigger mood swings, headaches, fatigue, irritability, and digestive issues—all symptoms that an MS patient really does not need. Diets that are too "on-and-off" simply will not work. Your goal is to use nutrition as medicine—as a form of treatment—which means that you have to side step the trap and reframe what food means to you.

What Dieticians Do Not Tell You About Dieting

A well-balanced diet has been key to healthy living since the early 1920s. Dieticians are often the people that you expect to approach when you have nutritional concerns and cannot get your questions answered by a doctor.

It is only logical to seek help from a licensed dietician—someone who has studied food and knows the ins and outs. Of course, many dieticians follow government prescribed programs. And this is where the trouble arises for patients with MS.

Most of the time, for a healthy human being, dieticians can do wonders. But sometimes when they work with MS patients, the wrong approach can lead to exacerbated symptoms. According to the Centre for Nutrition Policy and Promotion, the healthiest diet that you can eat is mainly made up of grain-heavy carbohydrates.

Then you should add servings of fruits and vegetables to your grains, even less protein and dairy products and sparingly eat fats, oils, and sweets.[39] In my experience, many dieticians base their diets on this idea of health, which is not ideal for patients with MS.

---

39   The Food Guide Pyramid, http://www.cnpp.usda.gov/publications/mypyramid/originalfoodguidepyramids/fgp/fgppamphlet.pdf

Certain foods seem to cause an allergic reaction in your body, which activates your immune system, causing an auto-immune attack and triggering MS symptoms. Many of these foods may be prescribed as part of your new diet that is supposed to make you healthier. However, the opposite can sometimes happen.

Not a single physician that I have seen throughout my life has ever suggested nutrition as a method of treatment. I have seen doctors in the USA and Latin America. My husband even had vascular dementia, and when I took him off gluten and increased his intake of healthy fats, his behavior changed dramatically to the point where I began weaning him off his medication.

My husband's doctors—similar to mine—could not understand his improvements, even after I told them what had caused it. They just looked at me like I had some kind of third eye. Clearly, it is easier to write a scrip than educate people on nutrition.

It is important that you are aware of the various types of food that trigger MS and the types of food that can help reduce MS symptoms. Here are some examples:

- There is growing evidence that consuming dairy or cow's milk is bad for MS patients.[40] The proteins in the milk are targeted by your immune cells because they mimic a part of your myelin sheath.
- Likewise, wheat and gluten[41] also trigger this immune response, which can provoke an MS attack. Interestingly, however, this is not the case in many warmer countries.

The Lifestyle Shift: It's Not a Diet

For patients with MS, there is no such thing as a quick fix diet that is going to solve their problems. Instead, you need to start thinking of

40   Fereshteh Ashtari, Cow's Milk Allergy in Multiple Sclerosis Patients, http://www.ncbi.nlm.nih.gov/pmc/articles/PMC3743324/

41   The MS Diet, http://www.msdietforwomen.com/ms-diet

food as medicine, which means that you have to make a real lifestyle shift from what you eat right now to healing foods.

A lifestyle shift is forever, which is the main difference between a diet change and a lifestyle revamp. The latest study by the University of Massachusetts has found that "the only consistent finding among the trials is that adherence—the degree to which participants continued in the program or met program goals for diet and physical activity— was most strongly associated with weight loss and improvement in disease-related outcomes."[42]

If you are committed to healing your Multiple Sclerosis, then it is a lifestyle intervention that you really need. That means following new rules and sticking to them.

- Find out which foods are best suited to your body, and develop a custom diet plan for yourself in conjunction with an open-minded dietician so that you can be happy with what you eat and still recover.

- Think about keeping a diet journal, where you can detail how you feel after you have eaten certain types of food. MS patients that do this sometimes realize it is food that triggers their attacks.

- Cut out harmful foods that damage your body, and seek out replacement foods that can enrich your eating experiences and still satisfy your need for different types of foods, flavors, and portions.

There will be some foods that you have to say goodbye to forever, but it is not as hard as you think. In fact, a month or so later you will not believe that you ever subjected your body to such large doses of carbohydrates, sugars, and dairy.

---

42   Dr Lisa Young, Lifestyle Intervention Beats Diet for Weight Loss: 6 Simple Changes to Make Today, http://www.huffingtonpost.com/dr-lisa-young/lifestyle-weight-loss_b_3831981.html

My Experience on the Macro Diet

The Macro Diet, or Macrobiotic Diet, was promoted as a potential healing diet for multiple sclerosis, so naturally I tested it out. Macrobiotics involves sea vegetables, brown rice, beans, and lots of whole grains.

The goal of the diet was to find a perfect balance for health and wellness. Some 40–60%[43] of the daily diet consists of organically grown whole grains like oats, rice, corn, and barley. Locally grown vegetables make up 20–30% of the diet, and 5–10% is reserved for beans like tofu, tempeh, miso, nori, and agar.

Eating cooked whole grains is a big part of the diet, instead of the unhealthy processed food choices that exist in grocery stores today. The Macro diet also advocates the absence of milk, with substitutions like broccoli, sesame seeds, and chickpeas[44] instead for calcium.

I was serious about testing it out, so I attended the Micho Kushi Institute in the United States for training and followed the diet for an entire year. My results were poor, and while I lost weight, my multiple sclerosis symptoms remained the same.

Later I realized that the sugar in all of the whole grains was preventing my body from healing. While this diet may work for people with very mild MS, I did not have success with it and therefore do not recommend it to people trying to recover from the disease.

The Macro Diet has some promising data, and I did all I could to learn about it while I used my body as a test vehicle. The results were clear to me—Macro did not work. It was back to the drawing board and on to a new type of nutrition to test out.

My Experience on the Raw Food Diet

My next adventure took me to the Raw Food Diet, another diet that was said to help people with MS. The goal for this diet was to stick

---

43   Macrobiotic Diet, http://www.webmd.com/diet/macrobiotic-diet

44   Milk and MS, http://www.macrobiotic.org/msmilk.html

to eating a lot of raw foods[45]—grains, vegetables, and fruits that are untouched by heat and therefore still contain lots of nutrients.

When you cook food, it can destroy the nutrients and enzymes there, and these are what your body needs to work well. While the Raw Food Diet definitely helps with weightloss because not many raw foods are high in calories, it was difficult to adhere to.

The diet restricts animal products so that can become an issue despite the nutritional boost that you get from the raw ingredients. During this diet, I had to eat uncooked, organic foods that were not processed, including nuts, greens, fruit, seeds, raw eggs, fish, and some unpasteurized dairy products.

I visited the Optimum Health Institute in San Diego, California, and the campus in Austin, Texas. I ate raw food and juiced for several days. There was a lot of wheatgrass involved. To be honest, complying with this diet was a hassle as it is very restrictive. I found it quite stressful and knew that there was no way to continue with it 100%. However, I did learn a thing or two there. To this day, I still blend raw green juice in the morning made mostly of fresh organic vegetables, which gives me a nutrient boost for the day.

All in all, the Raw Food lifestyle was not for me. I took elements from the experience and moved on to find my next potentially healing diet.

The Art of Dietary Restriction: Mindset Success

Even lifestyle shifts require restrictions of some kind. But when you dig into the restrictions, many of them are logical and easy to implement by changing your current habits. There is a subtle art to dietary restriction, and it starts with a revamped mindset.

- *Change your mindset.* Right now your beliefs are hampering your healing process. You might be eating junk food, and you might be solidly addicted to sugar. Whatever your result, it all

---

45   Raw Foods Diet, http://www.webmd.com/diet/raw-foods-diet

stems back to your mindset. Eating healthy foods means that your body will heal. That is the mindset to adopt.

- *Challenge your assumptions about food.* Knowledge is power, which means that if you conduct your own research into your current diet and what it is actually doing to your body, you may be a lot more inclined to change. Trans-fats, for example, are one type of food that will make you cringe when you read the data.

- *Release yourself of addictions.* Sugar is a huge addiction,[46] and based on recent studies, it is more addictive than cocaine. If you have struggled to stay on a diet in the past, it is because you failed to do a sugar detox. Try 28 days of no sugar! It changes your taste buds, your mindset, and the way that you feel about food.

- *Learn portion control.* I find that it is better to practice portion control with the right foods than restricting yourself. If you really feel like chocolate, for example, eat two blocks of low sugar, 90% dark chocolate. You can eat it every day after your detox to support a mainly sugar-free lifestyle.

Your mindset will really determine your success when it comes to making the necessary lifestyle changes that you need. Get used to the idea that good food means good for your body, not good for addiction, comfort, or emotional eating.

Testing Food Combinations for Results

Simplicity is always best when you begin to create your custom MS diet. I liked to try a new food for a few days and see how my body responded to it. Then I would test different combinations and see if I felt any better or any worse.

---

46   Dr Mark Hyman, Sweet Poison: How Sugar, Not Cocaine, Is One of the Most Addictive and Dangerous Substances, http://www.nydailynews.com/life-style/health/white-poison-danger-sugar-beat-article-1.1605232

It is the reason why I still juice vegetables because I find real value in the nutrients there. What you need to do is test what works best for you using the following processes.

Food combinations can cause all sorts of effects. As you are testing them, keep a food journal. Write down what your body feels like for review later on. Often combining the wrong foods can cause bloating, constipation, and all sorts of secondary issues.

I discovered that even if you eat a healthy diet, food combinations matter. That is why you should never over-eat and always chew your food properly and focus on food selections that are simple and easy to monitor for a few days.

Organize your meals into groups, and pair the best foods together. For a nutrient boost in the morning, get a juicer or make smoothies. Then eat something before lunch that tops you up and enjoy a proper lunch at the right time. Another snack and an early dinner give your body plenty of time to absorb the nutrients and relax.

Focus on the seven different food groups[47] first, and test them one by one. You will be surprised how quickly you can identify where your food issues lie. The food groups are: protein, starch, sugar, fat, fruits, vegetables, and non-starchy vegetables. Each of these has its place, and you need to find out where that place is on your daily menu.

My first step to recovery was nutritional information. Listen to other people's experiences, and build on them. Keep bio individuality in mind; we all respond differently to carbohydrates, proteins, and fats. You need to test them on yourself to feel what is best and what is not. Educate yourself first, then listen, then become a guinea pig —and finally, never give up. That is how I fine-tuned what I ate and dialed back my MS so much.

Make sure that your nutrition tests are conducted over a period of months, not days, or you will not experience any real change. When

---

47   Jo Jordan, How to Use Food Combining Techniques for Better Digestion, http://www. puristat.com/bloating/Food-Combining.aspx

I ate dessert every day, I had to take a nap in the afternoon. I would be exhausted by three in the afternoon. When I removed sugar from my diet, I could once again rise at six and go to bed at ten with no naps—a definite improvement.

Gluten is in so many processed foods that you could be eating it without even knowing it. That is why education always comes first. Eliminate all processed foods from your diet. You will feel a rapid change in your energy levels. My personal experience was that it lifted my brain fog, my mood improved, and my digestion healed itself. No gluten equals greater quality of life.

I firmly believe that you are able to create a diet plan for yourself that will help you reduce your MS symptoms. Be the super guinea pig for a while, and it will pay off for a lifetime!

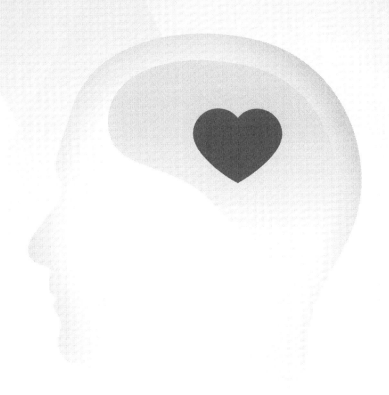

CHAPTER 7

Getting a Handle on Proper Nutrition

"Today, more than 95% of all chronic disease is caused by food choice, toxic food ingredients, nutritional deficiencies and lack of physical exercise."

MIKE ADAMS

For an individual with MS, few things are as important as nutrition when you have been left to treat your own disease. Getting a handle on the food that you are putting into your body will do wonders for your MS.

I have experienced a nutritional recovery and have spoken to many others who have also used food to heal. Figure out which foods match with your physiology, and you will take the first step to streamlining your diet and regaining your quality of life.

Smashing Through Modern Taboos

A taboo can be defined as a prohibited or restricted social custom. With multiple sclerosis patients, there is nothing more taboo than becoming extremely specific about the food you eat when doctors and medical science do not have solid rules on what works and what does not. People all around you may say that it is a waste of time.

When this happens, society tends to take the "nothing works" approach, which is incorrect. Just because there is no scientific data that adds up to a proven solution does not mean that you should not pursue your own nutritional solution.

If your sex drive fails you as an MS patient, that is a taboo that you need to speak about and find a solution for. Just like that instance, nutrition also needs to be considered as an overwhelmingly large part of your health that you control.

When your nutrition fails you, no one talks about it. They recommend little changes like "eat right" or "cut out fats," but they do not tackle the underlying cause—that food is not as healthy as it once was—and for the MS patient, this can cause pain, immobility, and exhaustion.

What You Don't Know About Food

Food is the fuel that makes up your body—you eat that cheese burger, and it becomes the fuel that is converted and becomes the cells and systems in your body. The saying is completely true that "you are what you eat."

What you do not know about food, however, may shock you. When I started digging beneath the taboos and discovering my own truths about food, I realized how in denial I really was about my diet and about food in general.

- Buy organic foods over conventional foods to improve your health.[48] They are more expensive than other types of food, but they do not contain growth hormones or antibiotics, and they contain fewer pesticides and higher omega 3 levels. In other words, these organic foods are naturally healthier for you than conventional food.

---

48   Tamar Haspel, Is Organic Better for Your Health? A Look at Milk, Meat, Eggs, Produce and Fish, http://www.washingtonpost.com/national/health-science/is-organic-better-for-your-health-a-look-at-milk-meat-eggs-produce-and-fish/2014/04/07/036c654e-a313-11e3-8466-d34c451760b9_story.html

- A diet low in saturated fat has had some positive results. In a study, it was found that MS patients that stayed on this low saturated fat diet experienced less deterioration than others.[49]
- A diet based mainly on processed foods is a killer for MS patients. These foods are brimming with artificial sweeteners, MSG, high fructose corn syrup, and chemical additives. These are bad for you, yes, but they also cause malnutrition because there is so little relevant nutritional value in the food.

By eliminating most (or all) processed foods, grains, and starches, you will instantly begin to experience a physical transformation. Instead of forcing your body to cope with bad foods, you will be giving your body healthy foods that aid in its repair and functioning.

What you do not know about food is that it has a much larger role to play in your health than science previously believed. Your choices matter. Where you shop matters. How you prepare your food matters, and how many nutrients you consume matters.

The Many Types of Food Quality on Sale

The mantra from the food industry has always been "there is no such thing as bad food, only bad diets," but they are only half right. There is no doubt that food quality plays an essential role in the diet of someone suffering with MS.

Not all food is created equal, which means that it is more important than ever to be educated about what you can and cannot do when it comes to your food choices. These will impact your health in ways you can only imagine.

Food quality is made up of several factors:

- *Where the food comes from and how it was grown, reared, or kept.* This refers to the free range eggs, the grass-fed beef, and

49   RL Swank, Effect of Low Saturated Far Diet in Early and Late Cases of Multiple Sclerosis, http://www.sciencedirect.com/science/article/pii/014067369091533G

fresh water fish debate. Buying food from batteries, where animals have been subjected to chemicals, modifications, and outright poor practices does affect the end product.

- *Manufacturers and food companies make false claims about nutrients in their food.* They purposefully keep things off their food labels and hide poor manufacturing practices with tricky word choices. For example, MSG, the famously bad additive, is also called hydrolyzed vegetable oil, which is downright misleading.

- Avoid all junk food and processed food. It lacks nutrition and is among the lowest quality food that you can eat. When you indulge in fast food, you are consuming things that could trigger your MS, along with so many GMO foods and other unhealthy chemicals, additives, fats, and sugars.

The good news is that you can shop for organic produce at your local farmers market or at another organic food shop. Buy locally, and buy fresh foods only. Get out of the habit of returning to fast food because it is cheap and easy. This kind of mentality will force you to struggle twice as hard with your body.

The Carbohydrate Conundrum

Carbohydrates are now the predominant element in our modern diets. There is no burger without a bun and fries. There is no steak or chicken without mash potatoes. All of our modern dishes revolve around carbohydrates as our central food source.

Everyone's MS is different, and there is no "one-size-fits-all" solution. But the latest research has uncovered that certain carbohydrates are quite bad for MS patients. Stated simply, any carb eventually becomes sugar in the body, but the carbs you choose to eat matter.

On one hand, you have the potato, breads, baked goods, pasta, wheat, and gluten conundrum. While carbs are meant to be a readily available source of energy for the human body, the high sugar content that develops into an addiction causes the over-consumption of carbs. This leads to fat gain and a much unhealthier situation for your body.

Sugar, as it stands, has been studied[50] and found to cause disability progression in MS patients. The more unhealthy carbohydrates you eat, the worse off you will be. I am not advocating the complete removal of carbs from your diet, but enough is enough! Grains and high starch foods should be used with care or not at all.

There is still a plethora of healthy carbohydrates to choose from, but they are vegetable-based. Sugar keeps your body in a state of ill-health, and it can trigger MS attacks if overused, like it often is in the modern diet. Balance your sugar levels,[51] keep them steady, and do not overindulge with carbs if you want to have a more stable body.

The point is that you will benefit from testing out lower carbohydrate foods and cutting out all of those carbs that cause weight gain and sugar addiction.

Gluten intolerance is a very real thing, and you should test for it. Get the blood tests; they do not cost that much, and they reveal a lot. If you are going to eliminate only two things from your diet, it would be gluten and sugar. They are in everything, and as a result, humans consume a lot of it. Sugar is the new cocaine of the health industry. It is hugely addictive and ruins the human body.

Sugar makes your body inflamed; I used to get so tired from eating it. Chronic conditions always revolve around inflammation, so it makes scientific sense to remove the cause of that inflammation so that your health improves.

Robert Lustig advocates that all calories are not created equally and that sugar is the worst thing to happen to people in many

---

50   Richeh Wael, The Association Between Serum Glucose Level and Disability Progression in Multiple Sclerosis, http://www.neurology.org/cgi/content/meeting_abstract/80/1_MeetingAbstracts/P04.130

51   Blood Sugar Balance and Multiple Sclerosis, https://www.theholisticdirectory.co.uk/articles/story/blood-sugar-balance-and-ms

years. Lustig called sugar the "villain" responsible for the obesity and chronic disease outbreak and says that sugar is added to 80%[52] of packaged foods. Sugar tends to hide in food and can appear on food labels in more than 40 different forms. You may believe you are avoiding it, but there is no real way to be sure because it is so unregulated.

It is essential to know how much sugar there is in food with clear package labels. Manufacturers mix it into everything to sell more products; even mayonnaise contains sugar. Sausages, salad dressing, and tomato ketchup have sugar in them. Natural or unnatural, people are eating way too much of it.

Sugar substitutes like Splenda have the same molecular reaction in your body, which means that they are the *same* as eating sugar. Do not replace sugar with anything except Stevia. It will be a challenge shopping for a sugar-free lifestyle, but the time is worth it. Cut out gluten and sugar as I have said to experience the wonder of natural health.

Working With Specific Types of Protein

Protein is essential in building the muscles in your body, among several other critical functions. For MS patients, this is a function that needs to work smoothly to reduce muscle pain and weakness. Back in the old days, people were told that eating red meat would cause saturated fat and cholesterol level overload, which would damage your health.

These days it has been found to be false and quite damaging to people that need red meat to perform vital functions like cell wall repair. The real truth is that you need a healthy balance of fats, namely polyunsaturated fat and Omega 3s and 6s to function well.[53]

---

52   Stephanie Schomer, The Sweet Lowdown: Exposing the Unhealthy Truth About Sugar, http://www.oprah.com/health/Health-Risks-of-Sugar-Robert-Lustig-Interview_1

53   Kristen Michealis, Healthy Meats: What to Buy, http://www.foodrenegade.com/healthy-meats-what-to-buy/

With meat these days, you have to watch out for hormone and antibiotic levels, how your meat is fed (GMO crops), and whether they are left to roam or are pumped full of growth hormones to get big while being unable to move. You need to buy specific types of healthy, ethically reared protein.

- Only choose grass-fed, pastured, free-range meat choices. It can be a better choice to buy in bulk directly from farmers to save on the costs, as these are the most expensive meats to buy.

- Buy organically reared meat that was raised without the use of antibiotics or hormones. Be careful of labels that use broad "organic" and "naturally raised" terms as these are often false and have nothing to do with the way the animal was raised. Also take care to avoid meats with additives, preservatives, nitrates, and nitrites.

For beans especially—an important protein—you have to watch out for how it was grown. Soy beans, for example, are a great source of protein,[54] but almost *all* soy crops in the U.S. are genetically modified. They are no longer healthy for human consumption.

Hydration and Your Body

Hydration is a concern for MS patients because if your body is dehydrated, it cannot absorb the vital nutrients it needs to function. And as you know, without nutrients, your MS symptoms and attacks will worsen.

For these reasons, it is important to drink at least two quarts of water a day[55] and to cut out heavy caffeine use. This will help with the common MS symptoms of constipation and bowel issues. Drinking enough water keeps your cells hydrated and cools your body.

---

54   Tom Philpott, Monsanto GM Soy Is Scarier Than You Think, http://www. motherjones.com/tom-philpott/2014/04/superweeds-arent-only-trouble-gmo-soy

55   Multiple Sclerosis, http://www.nytimes.com/health/guides/disease/multiple-sclerosis/lifestyle-changes.html

Even though much of the hype about being properly hydrated as an MS patient is unsubstantiated, I have found proper hydration essential in my own life. Perhaps you can test it out to see if water has been a missing element in your diet as well.

A hydrated body works better, communicates in a more effective manner, and does not have to divert resources because of dehydration. Even a 2% drop[56] in water levels in your body can cause dehydration. The fact is that most people walk around dehydrated without even knowing it.

Water should be consumed throughout the day, sipping on it as often as possible to avoid dehydration. Coffee and other beverages are not a substitute for pure water. Reports have come in about people with MS suffering with dehydration, so it is a problem that you might want to check out.

Hydration in the human body is key to overall health and wellness. If you cannot maintain your water levels, your body will react. For MS patients, this may cause some unpleasant side effects, so add water to your new lifestyle plan.

The Healthy Fats You've Been Avoiding

Fat has been demonized by the media and the medical industry for many years. Has your doctor ever told you to avoid animal fat or any fat at all because it would result in disease?

Years later, the people that avoided the fats still became sick with disease. This is because not all fats are bad for you, and some can actually rapidly improve the quality of life for MS patients. The healthy fats that you should be consuming are polyunsaturated fats and Omega 3s and 6s because they reduce inflammation, which helps with MS.[57]

---

56   Dehydration, http://www.ndhealthfacts.org/wiki/Dehydration

57   LR Mehta, Polyunsaturated Fatty Acids and Their Potential Therapeutic Role in Multiple Sclerosis, http://www.ncbi.nlm.nih.gov/pubmed/19194388

Foods like coconut oil and palm oil are packed with these Omegas and should become a part of your diet. By consuming fish, flaxseed, and other forms of readily available fats like these, your body will have the ingredients that it needs to reduce MS attacks.

Harvard recently published extensively[58] on this shift from "no fat" to "full fat." Saturated and trans fats are still bad for you, but most other kinds are desperately needed in your diet. These good fats are mainly found in vegetables and fish.

If you have been avoiding all forms of fat for years, this is the time to change. Your body needs fat to keep your brain healthy, which can insulate you against the neurodegenerative effects of MS. It is also important to point out that both bad fats that will harm you are constantly found in junk food and restaurant food.

Switch to olive oil, grass-fed butter, and coconut oil when you cook, and steer clear of other types of oil that allow large quantities of bad oils into your diet. Be mindful about where you eat and what oils they use to cook with.

I remember back in the '80s when everything was low fat to prevent heart disease and other chronic conditions. Scientific studies, however, have proved this line of thinking as incorrect. There are saturated fats that your body desperately needs, like coconut oil and medium chain triglycerides. My husband, who has vascular dementia, had a great lipid profile because he loved olive oil and ate a lot of it, but even then, when we included coconut oil, things improved at a central level. If you have brain fog, coconut oil is the right choice. I consume it myself to keep my brain healthy.

I conducted a brief study, taking my lipid profile prior to coconut oil, which saw my cholesterol oscillating over 200 with difficulties keeping my triglycerides down. Just last week, after months of consuming coconut oil, my total cholesterol is amazingly low, and

---

58   The Truth About Fats: Bad and Good, http://www.health.harvard.edu/fhg/updates/Truth-about-fats.shtml

my triglycerides are very, very low; my good cholesterol—HDL—is up, and my bad cholesterol—LDL—is down. That is proof to me. Do your own study within the period of 30 days, and you will see results.

We were wrong in thinking that all saturated fat was evil. They help control the inflammatory process in the body, enhance your immune system, and improve everything across the board when you consume good fats. Avoid vegetable oil and bad fats for best results.

Eating to Restrict Candida Growth

Candida is a yeast-based fungus that is found in the human body. It is usually benign and does nothing to harm your health. However, candida can grow out of control if left unchecked, and it has been linked with MS[59] in many ways.

Overgrowth of Candida is hard to treat and almost impossible to get rid of for patients with MS. Interestingly, it has been cited as a cause and ongoing problem for many people with MS. When Candida overtakes the body, it releases toxins that result in symptoms that can mimic the symptoms of MS.

Things like probiotics and antifungals can be used, but ultimately it is your diet that has caused the overgrowth. High sugar anything promotes the growth of Candida because it is a yeast that feeds on sugars. For this reason, you need to cut down on your sugar intake or stop eating sugar altogether.

Do this for a few weeks to see how you feel. If it works, then you know that many of your MS symptoms were directly related to a Candida overgrowth in your body, which is common. Avoid dairy, high sugar fruits, and any obvious sugar foods.

This means avoiding alcohol and any sugary beverages and switching to water with a small squeeze of lemon in it. It will not be easy, but if it basically takes away your MS symptoms, it is well worth the test.

---

59   What Causes Multiple Sclerosis?, http://www.holistichelp.net/blog/what-causes-multiple-sclerosis/

Because foods like coffee, sugar, and wheat products can promote the growth of Candida, it makes sense to test your diet free of these foods for a week or two. Studies[60] have proven that high Candida growth is directly associated with MS, so take it seriously.

Eating for Life: Inspiring Principles

Eating for life means so much more to an MS patient that has tried multiple diets and treatments and still finds themselves deteriorating. Remember that dieting does not work for MS or even for people that want to lose weight long term.

That is why this lifestyle intervention needs to happen. Follow these principles of eating for life, and you will improve the state of your MS. I cannot guarantee it, but I have lived through the experience myself and am functional and whole again.

- Find a diet that suits your body by testing different food combinations once you have eliminated all unhealthy food options from your diet forever. Begin with a 28-day sugar detox so that you can maintain your lifestyle change.

- You can cheat two days in every month so that deprivation does not get to you. But any more than this and you will slide back into worsening symptoms. Keep in mind that you are eating to stop MS and improve your life.

- Be consistent, and never allow your program to end. When you find a diet that works, stick to it. The longer you are on these diets, the better you feel. If you feel great after three months of eating right, do not stop! A year later, you will be a whole new person, but these interventions require commitment and real dedication.

- I have seen people who thought that they could not change their eating habits who have adopted these changes and

---

60   J Benito-Leon, Association Between Multiple Sclerosis and Candida Species: Evidence From a Case-Control Study, http://www.ncbi.nlm.nih.gov/pubmed/20556470

thrived. Anyone can do them, at any age, to experience the positive effects. Food is life, and you need to eat to keep yours healthy.

- Take note that non-gluten carbs like rice, potatoes, and pumpkin can have similar reactions in the body, almost the same as gluten. Stick to low carbohydrate vegetables only to repair your ailing immune system. Do not supplement with other carbs when you remove sugar and gluten from your diet.

I eat a lot of berries because they are low in sugar, and I eat a good amount of quality protein with a dominant order of fats. Salmon is rich in Omega 3s, and I only eat grass fed meat. I avoid farm raised fish that could contain heavy metals and stick to ocean fish.

If you want to learn more about curing MS with food, start with Dr. Terry Wahl, then move on to Dr. David Perlmutter with his book *Grain Brain*, then Dr. William Davis with his research on wheat bellies, Nora Gedgaudas on *Primal Mind, Primal Body*, and finally Tom O'Brian, who has done a lot of great work on gluten sensitivity and its reactions in the human body. It starts with knowledge!

Inspire yourself every day by keeping food in context. Get your family to make the diet shift as well so that it is easier for you. Do not allow anyone to make you feel bad for not eating bad foods, because they can trigger your MS.

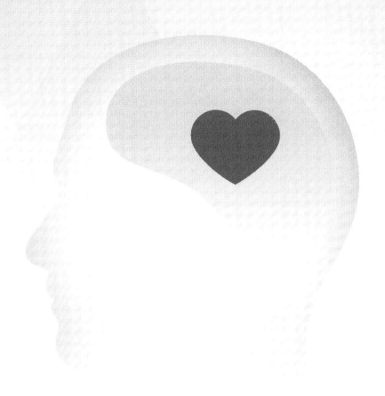

CHAPTER **8**

The Gluten Free Diet Explained

"Aside from some extra fiber, eating two slices of whole wheat bread is really little different, and often worse, than drinking a can of sugar-sweetened soda or eating a sugary candy bar."

WILLIAM DAVIS, WHEAT BELLY

I have already spoken about my experience with gluten and how cutting it out had such a drastic effect on my health and wellness. While the Macro Diet and the Raw Food Diet both taught me different things, ultimately they only mildly reduced my MS symptoms. It was not until I cut out gluten that I finally began to experience some form of recovery.

You may have noticed the craze circling the world right now as new research comes to light proving the many flaws in our modern diet. Gluten is one of the main culprits, and I have studied it extensively to educate you on why you should never eat it again.

What Is Gluten, and Why Does It Matter?

Gluten is most commonly found in wheat, rye, and barley products. As a food protein, it acts as the glue that gives food its shape and holds everything together. A survey from the NPD Group[61] recently claimed that some 30% of people in the U.S. either do not eat gluten or want to cut down on their gluten consumption.

Even more shocking are the climbing rates of gluten sensitivity and the research on how gluten might affect MS. Gluten consists of two types of protein: gliadin and glutenin.[62] Gliadin is generally the protein type that people respond negatively to, and it is in everything. Gluten in flour, for example, is what forms strong protein strands— like when you mix flour with water and the proteins create dough, which will rise when baked.

When certain individuals are sensitive to gluten, their immune systems attack it because it identifies the proteins as a foreign invader, like bacteria. I have personally found a gluten-free diet to be hugely beneficial, and Mr. Ashton Embry, founder of MS Direct,[63] also recommends that MS patients cut gluten grains out of their diet for improved health.

Gluten sensitivity is not the same as celiac disease, although many gluten-sensitive people benefit from dropping gluten from their diets altogether. With celiac disease, digesting gluten is problematic, and nutrient absorption is stunted. People with gluten sensitivity, however, do not have the disease even though they still experience adverse effects from gluten in their diet.

At the same time, the rate of celiac disease[64] is increasing, and if you have MS, the fatigue from gluten could be making things

---

61   Gluten-Free Diet Appeals to 30 Percent of Adults, Survey Says, http://www. huffingtonpost.com/2013/03/06/gluten-free-diet_n_2818954.html

62   Kris Gunnars, 6 Reasons Why Gluten May Be Bad for You, http://authoritynutrition. com/6-shocking-reasons-why-gluten-is-bad/

63   Donald A Ozello, MS and Gluten-Free Diet, http://www.livestrong.com/ article/239686-ms-gluten-free-diet/

64   Alberto Rubio-Tapia, Robert Kyle, Increased Prevalence and Mortality in Undiagnosed Celiac Disease, http://www.gastrojournal.org/article/S0016-5085(09)00523-X/abstract

significantly worse for you. Gluten sensitivity and non-celiac gluten sensitivity cause troubling symptoms for MS patients, which can make relapses worse and more frequent.

Research on Gluten Exposed

When your body is resistant to gluten, it struggles to break down the proteins that cause issues in your digestive tract. As you know, I am a solid believer in "healthy gut–healthy life" which I have found to be true by testing out different diets for myself.

By removing gluten from your diet, you give your body a better chance at keeping inflammation low. This reduction in inflammation allows your body to naturally repair itself better, your immune system functions more efficiently, and the nutrients you digest are absorbed with greater ease. Make sure that you avoid hidden gluten products, like oats. They do not contain gluten, but they are often contaminated with other gluten-containing grains.[65]

I firmly believe that eating well is the cornerstone to living well with MS. But with so much hype these days in the media, it is tough to know what to believe and what to ignore. The truth is that gluten does cause physical problems in your body, and you *do* feel better when you cut it out. However, doing this may not impact you the same way it impacted me.

Whether you believe it or not, I strongly suggest reviewing the evidence for yourself and testing the results in your own body. You can read all the facts, and when it comes down to it, if your body does not positively respond to the diet adjustment, then it means that gluten free will not benefit you. It really depends on your type of MS and how well you take care of yourself.

I recommend taking a 30-day period to remove gluten from your diet, and you should know for sure how gluten affects your MS.

---

65   Dr George Krucik, Gluten Allergies Food List: What To Avoid & What To Eat, http://www.healthline.com/health/allergies/gluten-food-list#2

People that have celiac disease will notice instantly improved health, and 80% of sufferers[66] do not even know they have it.

Why Gluten Free Works for MS

So where is the science proving that going gluten-free will work for MS patients? As I mentioned, there are arguments for and against gluten-free lifestyles. Multiple sclerosis causes your body to attack the myelin fatty substance that protects your nerves. This process is called demyelination, and it disturbs the nerve impulses traveling to and from your brain, reducing function and causing a host of other symptoms.

When you understand the relationship between symptoms and diet, you will better be able to control your health by reducing your symptoms via correct nutrition. A very big part of that is removing gluten from the equation. Patients with celiac disease (an autoimmune disease triggered by gluten) rapidly improve when they remove gluten from their diets.

Interestingly, in a 2001 study conducted by Kieslich,[67] patients that have celiac disease can also present with central nervous system abnormalities in an MRI. This proves that gluten-induced autoimmune disease can cause visible plaques in an MRI, much like MS—another autoimmune disease—does. That is enough cause to test the gluten-free diet.

You can very easily test to see if you are allergic to gluten grains. You can ask your doctor to test you for gluten sensitivity using a blood test. If necessary, you can also have further invasive studies using an endoscopy. Otherwise, all you have to do is cut out all forms of gluten for a few weeks to see if your health bounces back. If it

---

66   A Fasano, I Berti, Prevalence of celiac disease in at-risk and not-at-risk groups in the United States: a large multicenter study, http://www.ncbi.nlm.nih.gov/pubmed/12578508/

67   Donald A Ozello, MS and Gluten-Free Diet, http://www.livestrong.com/article/239686-ms-gluten-free-diet/

does, it means that gluten has been hitting the pause button on your healing process for too long, so remove it from your diet. I did, and I have never regretted it.

If I had continued on prescribed medication, I would be bedridden right now—of that I am positive. Restructuring your diet and removing food allergies can repair your digestive tract and, in so doing, help your body heal in ways you did not even realize it needed.

My research has led me to believe that a diet without gluten benefits an MS patient for some basic reasons. It reduces inflammation in your body, improves nutrient uptake, and facilitates healing, not to mention the medical connections between other autoimmune diseases that cause nerve damage.

Sources of Gluten in a Modern Diet

The good news is that gluten-free has taken the world by storm, which means that you can buy products free of gluten in most grocery stores and choose the gluten-free option at most restaurants now. The key is to educate yourself on the sources of gluten so that you are aware of what you are eating. Gluten can sneak into many foods and recipes, especially food prepared by others. If you are aware of the source, you can make the right decisions for yourself.

There are three big or dominant sources of gluten: wheat, rye, and barley. Wheat products include things like bread, freshly baked goods, pasta, soups, cereals, sauces, and salad dressings. You can nearly guarantee that if soup or sauce comes in a packet, box, or bottle, there will be gluten inside that product. It is very important to read nutritional labels before purchasing or consuming packaged products. Make it a healthy habit to do so.

Next is barley, which can be found in beers, malt vinegar, soup, food coloring, and malt. Finally, rye is located most often in bread, pasta, cereal, and rye-based beer. Aside from these products, you should also be wary of triticale,[68] which is a new kind of grain specifically grown to be similar to wheat. This also contains lots of gluten. Again, it is important to read nutrition labels. If you are not familiar with new food ingredients like triticale, then take time to research or make another choice. As a rule of thumb, do not eat food with ingredients you have never heard of.

Oats are another potential source of gluten. While oats are naturally gluten free, they are generally processed in facilities that also process foods that contain gluten. Therefore, many people with gluten sensitivities do not eat oats or only purchase gluten-free oat products.

There are a number of other items that include gluten of which you may be unaware. Did you know that soy sauce contains gluten? So does beer. Check out the list below for additional products.

Foods that contain gluten:

- Wheat bran
- Wheat germ
- White flour
- White whole wheat flour
- Graham flour
- Triticale
- Kamut
- Semolina
- Spelt
- Pasta
- Couscous
- Bread
- Flour tortillas

---

68   Triticale – All About Grains, https://www.usaemergencysupply.com/information_center/all_about_grains/all_about_grains_triticale.htm#.U9iBK_mSySo

- Cakes
- Cookies
- Sauces
- Dressings
- Cereal
- Crackers
- Oats
- Gravy
- Candy
- Imitation fish
- Malt
- Pastries
- Muffins/pancakes
- Soy sauce
- Salad dressing
- Lunch meat
- Hot dogs
- Matzo
- Seasoned rice[69]
- Foods that do not contain gluten (safe to eat!):
- Organic corn
- Rice (all forms)
- Amaranth
- Buckwheat
- Montina
- Millet
- Quinoa
- Teff

---

69   What Foods Have Gluten?, http://www.diabetes.org/food-and-fitness/food/planning-meals/gluten-free-diets/what-foods-have-gluten.html

- Sorghum
- Soy
- Milk
- Butter
- Margarine
- Real cheese
- Plain yogurt
- Canola oils
- Plain fruits
- Vegetables
- Meat
- Seafood
- Eggs
- Nuts
- Beans
- Legumes
- Flours made from beans and legumes
- Single spices
- Tapioca flour
- Potato starch flour
- Cornstarch
- Distilled vinegar
- Distilled alcoholic beverages[70]

I would also warn you against gluten substitutes. Just because something is gluten-free does not mean it is healthy. Gluten-free foods may still contain sugar, which leads to inflammation, as well as dense starches, like rice, corn, and potato, that quickly turn to

---

70   The Basic Diet (What I Can Eat), http://www.glutenfreeliving.com/nutrition/the-basic-diet/

sugar in the body. The key is to know what you are eating and to make better choices. There are lots recipes for gluten-free, low-carb bread, for example, that do not contain sugar or dense starches and are made with almond flour, coconut flour, and flaxseeds. Take a look online for ideas.

The Leaky Gut

Individuals with a leaky gut experience symptoms like joint pain, fatigue, digestive problems, insomnia, low libido, and depression. It is a condition that affects the lining of the small intestine when it becomes damaged, causing indigested food particles, toxic waste products, and bacteria that leak into your blood stream through your intestinal wall.

These cause a serious autoimmune response in your body, causing inflammation, allergic reactions to food, and a host of additional symptoms. But the worst damage from leaky gut comes from the fact that your intestines do not produce enough enzymes to digest your food correctly. Nutrient absorption becomes difficult, and hormone imbalances result.

This weakened immune system is wide open and can cause many other diseases or disorders.[71] It is caused and exacerbated by dairy, soy, sugar, caffeine, and the biggest of all—gluten. To recover from a leaky gut—and reverse your negative immune system response—cut out these foods. The starch and sugar mix common in the modern diet will make your MS much, much worse because of disorders like leaky gut syndrome and autoimmune responses to these foods.

Living Gluten-Free: How to Shop

Living gluten-free in a gluten-obsessed world is difficult. Because gluten hides in lots of different products, a balance needs to be struck

---

71 Your Gut and Autoimmune Disease, http://terrywahls.com/your-gut-and-autoimmune-disease/

between what you look for to avoid and the foods that you buy to make up for the nutrient and caloric deficit. First of all, you cannot replace all of your gluten foods with "gluten-free" substitutes.

"Gluten free"' is a new sales tactic, just like "fat free" was 20 years ago. The industry is still up to its old tricks, with many gluten-free products containing nearly no nutritional value, and they are highly processed, which makes them automatically terrible for your health. You must avoid all processed foods, or it may exacerbate your MS.

That means when you go shopping, you will have to get into the habit of reading all of your food labels. Only shop for fresh fruits and vegetables and quality, grass-fed protein. Avoid grain-fed meat, or you will be eating gluten in your meat! Throw away your cheap vegetable oil, condiments, and other gluten-rich items.

When you move away from gluten, you will also have to compensate by eating more fresh foods to keep your nutrition levels up. With your main carbs gone, you will be hungry—so buy more fresh foods, and get into the habit of making these vegetables the base of every meal so that you do not miss the gluten so much.

Shop for more fresh food and fewer gluten-free products, and read your labels to make sure that gluten is not hiding in anything. Even a crouton's worth of gluten can cause reactions in your body, and it is easy to get that in from strange sources in your average day.

What Can and Can't You Eat?

You will need to discover for yourself the specifics of what you can and cannot eat. As a rule, all gluten products contain sugar, which means that they are highly addictive. You may struggle to get off them in the beginning because of your sugar dependency. Stick it out for 14 days of sugar-free struggle, and going without will feel a lot better.

- Gluten excludes all of your grain foods from your diet. But you should also look at limiting your intake of corn, as it is mainly genetically modified, and rice because it is a heavy carbohydrate that contains lots of sugar.

- Gluten is often found in fast food or junk food, processed food, and spices, so decide now to never go to another fast food restaurant again; it will only make your MS worse. Instead, switch to the occasional gluten-free pizza or a high protein and vegetable replacement from a better quality restaurant that is not about fast food.

- You can, however, eat as many fresh vegetables as you like and limited fruits—especially the low sugar kind like berries and strawberries. Focus on butter over margarine, eat plenty of fresh fish and seafood (no battery fish), and always buy free range, grass fed meat products.

- Wine in limited quantities can be consumed to keep your sugar levels down, but you should avoid sugar-rich alcohol like spirits, or gluten-rich alcohol like beer. As a rule, you should also cut out all sugary juices and choose to stick to tea, coffee, smoothies, and water or fruit-infused water.

- Never eat canned foods, as they are processed and contain harmful chemicals, not to mention preservatives that are unnatural for the human body. Fresh is always best, and organic is even better.

If you are going to eat to live—as someone who is recovering from MS—you need to be strict and consistent with your food choices. There is no point in staying away from gluten one day and then eating two pizzas the next day. Food matters to your health.

The Gluten Danger Zone: Substitutes

The "gluten free" fad is just that—a diet craze that will come and go like the Atkins diet or the South Beach diet. For you as an MS patient, you will be cutting out gluten as a medical lifestyle choice so that your health improves. I strongly believe that if you do, you will experience greater health and add years to your life.

That said, it can be easy to fall into bad habits. We all love carbs, which is why they make up most of the modern diet. Before, when human ate less carbs, we had lower disease rates and were healthier overall as a species. Now advertising has changed that. Large groups of people are lied to about food, and they do not bother to find out what the lie is about.

Gluten substitutes can be dangerous for a few very relevant reasons. An entire new industry is popping up around this fad, which means that a lot of bad food is going to be sold to people that believe it is a healthier option, when it may not be. The truth is that many gluten-free products lack fiber, and you need this for good digestive health.

There are also way too many carbohydrates in gluten-free products, meaning that they contain loads more starch to compensate for the lack of gluten—and where there is starch, there is sugar. As you know, sugar is horrifying for your body.

Many of these newly styled "healthy" foods are crazy expensive, by a margin of about 242%[72] according to the U.S. National Library of Medicine, which makes them hard to maintain. Gluten-free products are also stuffed with calories, and they can make you gain weight—instead of losing weight to help your MS symptoms.

You will find that many of these products have no nutrients, because they are "bad" carbs, and the xanthan gum used can cause similar digestive distress—even resulting in diarrhea if you eat too much of it. In other words, you cannot simply go gluten-free; you have to cut out gluten and adopt a healthier way of eating to heal.

---

72   L Stevens, Gluten-free and Regular Foods: A Cost Comparison, http://www.ncbi.nlm. nih.gov/pubmed/18783640

Living With Someone Who Eats Gluten

By now, you may be realizing what a challenge this lifestyle conversion will be. It becomes even more difficult when you consider that you will be living in a home with other people who will continue to eat gluten, which may corrupt your diet. On a very serious note, it would benefit your entire family to remove gluten, sugar, and heavy carbs from their diet.

You should consider sitting down with your family and adjusting your eating habits as a whole. Otherwise, there is a good chance that you will never fully be able to get off carbs or gluten, which means that you will never have the quality of life you deserve.

If your family is not willing to be unified with you in this adjustment, then you will have to think outside the box. I suggest two different fridges to keep you motivated and away from the foods that you will crave but should not eat.

When you go shopping, it will become important for you to prioritize eating your gluten-free foods over others, so you will end up with two shopping lists. This can get confusing, and it often leads people to fall back into bad habits. Plus, with the fatigue from MS, you will need all of the support and help that you can get.

Do not expect your family to be happy about it, but take the time to explain that the adjustment will improve your quality of life and that medical research supports the shift for everyone. If you approach the diet as a family, it becomes exciting and doable. When you go at it alone, you do have to assume responsibility for what you eat.

Tell everyone around you that you are no longer eating gluten or anything with sugar in it. No more hot dogs brought from work, no more doughnut treats. You must not be given the opportunity to indulge. It becomes easier if you limit this temptation by getting your family and friends on board.

Living with someone who eats gluten is fine if you watch what you eat and cook for yourself. If not, you will need to get creative to stay on course—for the good of your MS.

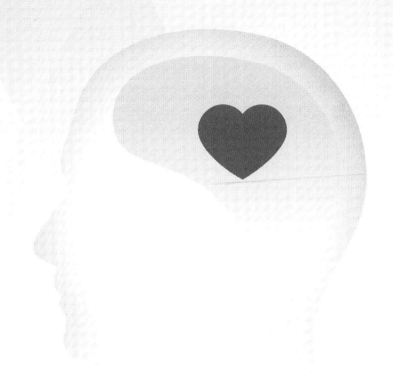

CHAPTER 9

Medical Research on Gluten and Diet

*"I've had plenty more patients come through my doors
and leave with a pain-free head, thanks to the adoption
of a gluten-free diet."*

DAVID PERLMUTTER, GRAIN BRAIN[73]

While the research on gluten remains inconclusive with varied results, it is clear that in specific patients with MS, cutting gluten out of their diet can have long-lasting effects. This means that a gluten-free diet has the potential to drastically reduce your MS symptoms, providing you with a better quality of life than you are currently living with.

Medical research on gluten is split in half—those for gluten and those against it. Many studies are funded by food companies, and you have to be careful of that. So far, the research I have read was convincing enough for me to try it, and as you know, I was fortunate enough to almost obliterate my MS symptoms.

Three Studies on Gluten and MS

There are three main studies that convinced me of the efficacy of testing out a gluten-free diet.

---

73   Grain Brain Quotes, https://www.goodreads.com/work/quotes/24064606-grain-brain-the-surprising-truth-about-wheat-carbs-and-sugar--your-b

The Annals of the New York Academy of Sciences conducted a study[74] to see if gluten sensitivity in multiple sclerosis was a myth or a clinical truth. The results were clear: The scientists discovered gluten antibodies in 98 MS patients, and these were significantly higher than their control groups.

The conclusion was that while these antibodies need to be studied further to establish a relationship with MS, a gluten-free diet should be considered in specific cases with patients that have these antibodies.

Another study, conducted by the Royal Hallamshire Hospital in the UK,[75] found that antigliadin antibodies were not only a marker for celiac disease but for people with many other neurological disease like MS, even if they do have normal small bowel mucosa.

Finally, another study by Acta Neurologica Scandinavica[76] also tested MS patients for responses to the antibodies generated in the body against gluten. They concluded that some proteins uptake is increased in MS patients compared to controls. All of this evidence gave me a direct path to investigating the link between MS and gluten even further.

The Link Between Celiac Disease and MS

Both celiac disease and multiple sclerosis are autoimmune diseases. At first glance, I did not think much of it, but after coming across more research, the ties became clear. If gluten can damage the

---

74   Dana Ben-Ami Shor, Gluten Sensitivity in Multiple Sclerosis, http://onlinelibrary. wiley.com/doi/10.1111/j.1749-6632.2009.04620.x/abstract?deniedAccessCustomisedMess age=&userIsAuthenticated=false

75   M Hadjivassiliou, A Gibson, Does Cryptic Gluten Sensitivity Play a Part in Neurological Illness? http://www.thelancet.com/journals/lancet/article/PIIS0140-6736(96)90540-1/abstract

76   K Reichelt, D Jensen, IgA Antibodies Against Gliadin and Gluten in Multiple Sclerosis, http://onlinelibrary.wiley.com/doi/10.1111/j.1600-0404.2004.00303.x/abstract?d eniedAccessCustomisedMessage=&userIsAuthenticated=false

nervous system in patients with celiac disease, could it do the same or even worsen the existing nerve damage in MS patients?

Research published in a 2011 study[77] shows a link between both diseases. Spanish clinicians analyzed the prevalence of positive celiac blood tests and biopsies in people with confirmed MS and in their first degree relatives. There were 72 MS patients, 126 relatives, and 123 controls. The results were very revealing.

The study determined that celiac disease was found in 11.1% of MS patients compared to 2.4% of the control subjects. Even more shocking was the first degree relative results, which showed a 32% prevalence in close relatives. Every single MS patient that was placed on a gluten-free diet improved considerably.

These improvements involved both gastrointestinal and neurological improvements—meaning that cutting out gluten reduced their MS symptoms significantly. While there is still a lack of research on how celiac disease and MS are related, one thing is certain. If you are, like many MS patients, sensitive to gluten, removing it from your diet will instantly help you.

Correlations between MS and gluten intake have led to many studies; one in particular[78] resulted in findings that concluded all MS patients with gastroenterological complaints should get tested for celiac disease, as the prevalence is higher than normal. In these instances, MS patients would benefit from avoiding gluten at all costs.

How Salt Affects MS Patients

Sugar has already gone wild and now salt, too? Unfortunately, this may be the case. Salt could be the reason that immune systems are turning against people, a recent study suggests. BBC News Health

---

77   Jane Anderson, Celiac Disease and Multiple Sclerosis, http://celiacdisease.about.com/od/symptomsofceliacdisease/a/Celiac-Disease-And-Multiple-Sclerosis.htm

78   HZ Batur-Caglayan, C Irkec, A Case of Multiple Sclerosis and Celiac Disease, http://www.ncbi.nlm.nih.gov/pmc/articles/PMC3556850/

reported on a team of scientists that have all gotten together to expose salt as a potential disease aggravator.

As it turns out, salt activates a part of the immune system that can target the human body. Your body's natural defense against infection is corrupted by the digestion of excess salt, which is now in more food products than ever before.

Salt has already been demonized by the medical community for causing hypertension, heart disease, and stroke, and the average American consumes volumes of salt in bread and cheese, where it hides. Some 90% of sodium[79] is consumed as salt, while 77% of a person's intake comes from processed or restaurant food, 6% from cooking and 5% that is added afterwards.

When a team of MIT and Harvard researchers[80] investigated how T-helper 17 cells were created—resulting in autoimmune disease—they discovered that a gene that is usually used to increase salt uptake in the gut was responsible. Mice were fed high salt diets and became more likely to develop diseases close to MS.

While a lot more research needs to be conducted on the link between salt and MS, it is advisable to switch to a low sodium salt or a Himalayan salt, which contains a lot of minerals that help you digest your food.

With salt becoming yet another reason to carefully monitor what you eat and where, MS patients should take action to reduce their sodium intake, in my opinion, or at least test it out to see if any physical benefits result from a three-month suspension of consuming lots of salt.

How Sugar Affects MS Patients

Refined foods contain a lot of sugar. In fact, if you look around the grocery store, it is hard to land on a product that does not contain

---

79   Salt Stats, http://www.cdc.gov/salt/pdfs/salt_stats_media.pdf

80   James Gallagher, Salt Linked to Immune Rebellion in Study, http://www.bbc.com/news/health-21685022

high sugar levels. And there are good reasons for this; namely, money. When sugar is added to food, it sells in higher quantities.

Sugar, unfortunately, has received a terrible reputation as being an MS patient's worst nightmare, and through my own tests and studies, I have found this to be true. One study, conducted by the Louisiana State University Health Sciences Center,[81] concluded that there is a direct correlation between MS disease progression and your blood glucose levels.

Refined sugar is especially bad and causes serious inflammation in your body. This inflammation does not get a chance to heal itself, as your blood sugar levels are constantly spiked from your modern diet of carbs and treats.

The quicker sugar can make it into your blood stream, the faster it will cause a flood of insulin into your body, which transcends the blood–brain barrier and affects everything from your cognitive function to the way your body processes food.

Sugar has a distinctly negative affect on your digestive system, which as you know, is important if you are going to reduce your MS symptoms. Even worse than sugar is artificial sweetener, which does the same thing in larger amounts as they are metabolized even faster by the body.

White sugar, and indeed all refined sugars, slows down your body's ability to absorb nutrients and function efficiently. When you have MS and your digestive system impacts your symptoms so much, you cannot afford to be malfunctioning in that department. I highly recommend removing sugar from your diet immediately.

Gluten, Wheat, and Sugar: Eliminate It Now!

After all of this research, it is safe to conclude that eating sugar,

---

81   Wael Richeh, Amparo Gutierrez, The Association Between Serum Glucose Level and Disability Progression in Multiple Sclerosis, http://www.neurology.org/cgi/content/meeting_abstract/80/1_MeetingAbstracts/P04.130

wheat or gluten of any kind should be carefully considered by an MS patient. I have lived without these foods in my life for many years without any further MS aggravations.

If you are anything like me, you will not only benefit from removing these foods but your entire life will change. Leaky gut is often caused by excesses of this potent combination. Leaky gut syndrome, as I mentioned earlier, results when the lining of your intestine becomes porous to food, which causes a host of symptoms—like bacteria overgrowth and intestinal issues. Modern medicine often focuses on treating the symptoms instead of the cause. But with the rise of functional medicine comes a new approach to health that looks for causes rather than just treating symptoms.

To give up sugar, know where it is hiding!

- Ketchup
- Baloney
- Fish Sticks
- Peanut Butter
- Soy milk
- Sports drinks
- Spaghetti sauce
- Added sugars show up in ¾ of all food in your local grocery store.

To recognize sugar on food labels, look for these misleading names:

There are 56 different names for sugar on food labels!

Barely malt, Barbados sugar, Beet sugar, Brown sugar, Buttered syrup, Cane juice, Cane sugar, Caramel, Corn syrup, Corn syrup solids, Confectioners' sugar, Carob sugar, Castor sugar, Date sugar, Dehydrated cane juice, Demerara sugar, Dextran, Dextrose, Diastatic malt, Diatase, Ethyl maltol, Free flowing brown sugars, fructose, Fruit juice, Fruit juice concentrate, Galactose, Glucose, Glucose solids,

Golden sugar, Golden syrup, Grape sugar, HFCS (high fructose corn syrup), Honey, Icing sugar, Invert sugar, Lactose, Malt, Maltodextrin, Maltose, Malt syrup, Mannitol, Maple syrup, Molasses, Muscovado, Panocha, Powdered sugar, Raw sugar, Refiner's syrup, Rice syrup, Sorbitol, Sorghum syrup, Sucrose, Sugar (granulated), Treacle, Turbinado sugar, and Yellow sugar.[82]

I believe that when you eliminate gluten, wheat, and sugar from your diet for longer than three to six months, it will reshape your body and kick start your healing capacity. This trifecta causes serious bowel inflammation, among other concerns. Droves of people across the globe are realizing how sick they have felt from things like "wheat belly" and "grain brain."

- Grain brain is a concept created by Dr. David Perlmutter that states most grains in the modern diet are responsible for neurologically degenerative disease like Alzheimer's and dementia. Cutting them out reduces your chances of age-related neurological damage. In MS patients, I also believe that it reduces cognitive issues.

- Wheat belly is a concept created by Dr. William Davis that speaks[83] about how carbohydrates, especially wheat, cause insatiable appetite and cycles of addiction to this food type that in turn invokes lifelong weight gain and illness.

Keep in mind that everyone is different. If you find you need more carbohydrates[84] in your diet, then work them in. But I strongly suggest you alter your diet immediately to begin benefitting from

82   TED Talks, Sugar: Hiding in Plain Sight – Robert Lustig, https://www.youtube.com/watch?v=Q4CZ81EmAsw

83   Kerry Shaw, Why Wheat Is Ruining Your Life: The Author of Wheat Belly Explains, http://www.mindbodygreen.com/0-9484/why-wheat-is-ruining-your-life-the-author-of-wheat-belly-explains.html

84   Kris Gunnars, The Sugar Free, Wheat Free Diet, http://authoritynutrition.com/the-sugar-free-wheat-free-diet/

improved nutrients and less inflammation. The proof will always be in the way that you feel. Test it for yourself.

The Desolation of Your Body: Grain Research

Many MS patients like myself grew up on grains and legumes, but the latest research warns us against continued consumption as they may be worsening our symptoms. While everyone is different, the truth remains that grain seems to be causing some harm in the bodies of MS patients. Not only have I experienced this for myself but I have seen it in others as well.

Grain is catastrophic for your body. Dr. Cordain claims[85] that the lectins from grains, tomatoes, and legumes help activate your T cells, which causes the negative immune response. Many of the lectins cling to receptors that can pass through the intestinal wall, or they hitch a ride on protein fragments derived from food.

Once past your gut, these lectins can activate your myelin-sensitive T cells via molecular mimicry. Lectins also cause the upregulation of proteins associated with the blood-brain barrier, which facilitates the entry of the activated T cells into your central nervous system, where they then attack your myelin. The daily intake of grains constantly places you at risk.

Moderate rice consumption is better for a person with MS than eating grains or any foods that contain these proteins, like tomatoes and legumes. By cutting out the grain, you will repair your leaky gut so that they will never reach circulation and will not have the chance to activate your T cells or attack your myelin.

If you take this theory of Dr. Cordain's to heart, you quickly realize how eating grain could play a significant role in theh combination of factors that are provoking your MS. As part of the Colorado State University team, Dr. Cordain is teaching this theory all over the

---

85   Ashton Embry, The Role of Lectins From Grains and Legumes in the MS Disease Process, http://www.direct-ms.org/sites/default/files/Lectins%20and%20MS.pdf

country. So far, there have been many positive responses and success stories.

The Paleo Diet and MS

The Paleo diet is very popular these days for weightloss. Closely related to the Mediterranean diet, the Paleo diet was created by Dr. Loren Cordain and is based on the fundamental principle that everyone is different and should eat according to their unique genetics.

But beyond that, all humans should eat like we used to in the old days, thousands of years ago, when all we had access to was fresh vegetables, fruits, meat, and limited grain. The Paleo diet is based on higher protein intake (like the hunter–gatherers of yesteryear), lower carb intake, high fiber, and moderate to high good fats consumption.

Dr. Terry Wahls beat multiple sclerosis after being on conventional medication for seven years and finally switching to the Paleo diet. Her theories led her to investigate mitochondria in the human body after realizing that brain shrinkage happens in many autoimmune diseases.

She was rapidly declining until she began to treat herself with nutrition. For her mitochondria to function correctly, she discovered that she needed more animal-based Omega 3s, creatine, and coenzyme Q10. She added them to her diet, and her deterioration slowed. But she wanted to recover, so she adopted the Paleo way of living.

After changing her eating for nine months, she went on an 18-mile bike ride![86] Like me, Dr. Wahls searched high and low for a solution and discovered it in something as simple as nutrition and adopting a new lifestyle. Elements of the Paleo diet may work for

---

86   Doctor Reverses Multiple Sclerosis in 9 Months By Eating These Foods, http://articles.mercola.com/sites/articles/archive/2011/12/23/overcoming-multiple-sclerosis-through-diet.aspx

you, so I suggest that you look into it.

Any diet that advocates the use of more animal-based Omega 3s, vegetables, fruit, and grass-fed protein sounds good to me. But it has to be used in conjunction with improved exercise and the ability to avoid the food triggers that we have spoken about. It is hard to adjust your eating habits but very worth it when your symptoms vanish.

The Power of Vegetables for MS

Vegetables are an essential part of a symptom-crushing MS diet. Myelin insulates your nerves in the central nervous system of your body, and it needs specific nutrients to function effectively; namely, the B vitamin group.

You also need sulfur and lots of good micro nutrients to keep your immune system healthy. When you do this, your body will have everything it needs to keep you stable, and you may not have another attack if you eat this way consistently.

- Eat lots of green leafy vegetables; these are rich in minerals and essential vitamins like A,C, K, and B. Consume at least one bag of leafy greens every day.
- Focus on getting enough iodine in your diet from seaweed, and eat a lot of brightly colored vegetables to take in antioxidants to balance out your free radical production.
- Include sulfur-rich vegetables like onions, mushrooms, asparagus, and cabbage to make sure that your body is working well.

Making sure that your body gets in enough nutrients will help you maintain good health. In some of the most remote areas in the world—where they are still eating fresh foods—these people consume three to ten times more than their recommended daily nutrient allowance. This ensures that they have the building blocks they need so that they never get sick.

You can do something similar by juicing. I juice mostly vegetables every morning to condense all of those great raw vegetables into something tasty and nutritious. It is a far better start than any cereal ever was because it genuinely makes me feel healthy and raring to go.

Dr. Terry Wahls[87] suggests that you find a way to consume nine cups of vegetables every day to get in the nutrients that you need. Think of a plant—if it does not get enough water and essential nutrients, it will become diseased. People are the same!

A Typical Alternative MS Diet Plan

A typical alternative MS diet plan would be very different to the food groups that you are used to eating. At first, it will seem like there is nothing "good" left to eat. But that is a misconception and your raging sugar addiction talking. Food actually tastes better once you have cut out sugar and wheat, which I found dulls the taste buds.

- Switch to grass-fed, not grain-fed, free range meats. Keep your red meat consumption at a reasonable level, and think about consuming organ meats like liver and kidney for additional vitamins, minerals, and CoQ10.

- Eat more raw foods, especially vegetables and fruit—least nine cups of veggies—and stick to low sugar fruits like berries.

- Wild fish and other ocean-reared fish are great for Omega 3s, and you can use natural herbs, lemon, and stock sauces to reduce gluten and sugar content.

- Consider investing in a juicer. About 30% of my diet is raw food, and I drink fresh vegetable juice almost every morning.

- Begin to consume more good fats like the ones found in coconut oil and extra virgin olive oil. Cut out canola oil, vegetable oil, and margarine forever.

---

87 Terry Wahls, Vegetables, http://terrywahls.com/tag/vegetables/

Your daily meal plan should be: juicing in the morning or eating eggs with a full plate of salad. Lunch should involve lots of vegetables, some fruit, a protein source, and a healthy serving of good fats. For dinner, this same model should be repeated in higher quantities. You decide what you like and how you should cook it.

Do not forget to take what you drink into account. No sugar-based drinks of any kind, ever. That means learning to enjoy coffee and tea without sugar or switching to a natural sweetener like Stevia. NuNaturals is my favorite brand because of the taste.

Embrace water, infused water, and juices that you make from fresh veggies. Cut out fruit juice and other artificial juices.

How to Customize Your Plan

Eating is a very personal pursuit. While you may not feel particularly influenced or changed by your food choices now, believe me, they make up how your body functions. Years of exposure to grain, junk food, and processed, frozen rubbish has impacted you. To customize your plan, I suggest working through the following stages.

Stage 1: Carbohydrate and sugar detox. Eat anything you like as long as you do not eat anything (I mean it) with sugar, wheat, or gluten in it. Go high carb-free for two weeks, and detox off sugar. You will withdraw, and it will feel horrible. That is when you know you are helping your body out. After two weeks, eat low carbs only. These include your starchier vegetables.

Stage 2: If you suspect a food group or item may be negatively impacting you, conduct personal food tests in three-month increments. Eliminate that food from your diet for a few weeks, and write down how you feel. At the end of the test, review the data. If you feel better without that food, cut it out.

Stage 3: Create your own MS busting diet with lots of Paleo/Mediterranean influence to guide your menu choices. Start to search for food based on healing and not attachment to food. Search online for recipes that are quick to prepare and only require a few ingredients rather than ones that require hours of waiting when you are hungry.

Stage 4: Prepare to be healthy. Precook foods and keep them in the fridge. A roast chicken leg is great to pull out for lunch with some leafy greens and vegetables. Work on expanding your fresh food menu so that you do not get bored of eating the same things.

Stage 5: Recover and maintain! During this process, keep a list of the dishes that you enjoy, and recreate them. Get into the new rhythm of being healthy and recovering by ramping up your exercise regimen if you can.

As always, keep your eyes on the medical research online. I am sure in the coming years there will be many new findings about beneficial food choices for people recovering from MS! You should be the first to hear about it.

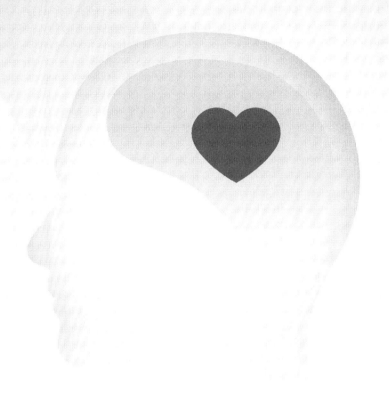

CHAPTER **10**

Cultivating a Self-Care Lifestyle

"Rest and self-care are so important. When you take time to replenish your spirit, it allows you to serve others from the overflow. You cannot serve from an empty vessel."

ELEANOR BROWN

Self-care is about understanding the challenges that your body faces and assuming responsibility for them. You need to make the choice to put yourself first after your MS diagnosis. Sometimes it is better to say no and know your limitations than to risk triggering your MS or allowing your health to deteriorate.

Self-care was not a priority for me or part of my lifestyle, which was largely because of my workaholic tendencies. I worked all day, travelled to lectures, was out the house nearly each night, and never took time out for myself. I always put my family first as I was the breadwinner.

How to Respond to Drug Treatments

In honesty, I did not practice self-care until I received my MS diagnosis. Even then, I did not do it until I worked through the denial phase. Today I make time to take care of myself and my own personal needs. I get massages, I eat correctly, I exercise, and I have learned to say no. As a people pleaser, this was not an easy lesson to learn.

The first thing you need to know about self-care is how to respond to drug treatments. There is a good chance that you are on medication and that you will use more than one kind during your MS journey. Knowing how to review the side effects and make an educated decision is key to the concept of self-care. If you do not know what might happen, you cannot spot it.

- Before a single chemical has passed your lips, follow this safety protocol. First ask your doctor about the side effects. Take note of what they say. Then read the package insert thoroughly. Finally, conduct 25 minutes of online medical research and 25 minutes of user review research.
- Use credible medical websites like Rxlist.com, Webmd.com, Drugs.com, and brand websites like Copaxone.com.[88] Make sure that you plug in the correct keyword as you search, and compare what the brand website says with what the others say.
- Your 25 minutes of medical research will be done on these sites. Then you will spend another 25 minutes researching how other MS patients found the drug. Record any potential side effects, and look out for them as you use the drug.

Check on your doses, contra-indications, reviews, and what critics say about these drugs.

Understanding the Pill-Consequence Principle

The pill-consequence principle warns people about the ease of popping pills to solve any ache or pain. When you have MS and a host of weird symptoms flare up, drugging them away or doing something similar can end up with severe consequences.

---

88   What Dose Is Right For You?, https://www.copaxone.com/about-copaxone/dosage-information

All medication has side effects, whether they are positive or negative. This includes over-the-counter medication, prescription drugs, or natural and herbal supplements. You will be taking a few medications if that is the route you choose, which means that you will regularly be consuming specific chemicals that could inflict long-term damage on your body and even activate secondary and tertiary diseases or conditions.

With MS symptoms, pain can become problematic, which leads to the use of over-the-counter painkillers. Muscle relaxants work for anxiety and ticks, and steroids are used as a type of treatment to prevent disease progression. You might take ginseng for energy because of your fatigue.

Even though all of this medication is varied—some conventional, some natural—all drugs have a consequence in your body. And that is really what the pill–consequence principle is about. As a person with MS, you need to make sure that you control your intake of medication, or you could end up with liver, kidney, and various other concerns.

For me, if I had known that my MS drug would cause gutters in my body, I would have thought twice about using it. You are now predisposed to needing more medication than many other people, so be wise about the choices that you make.

At all times, your medicine benefit needs to far outweigh the cost of the side effects.[89] If at any time they do not and the side effects become overwhelming, immediately contact your doctor and discuss alternatives.

Keeping Up With Modern MS Research

There are many ways that you can keep up with the latest MS research. You do not even have to purposefully go to the computer and search

---

89   Side Effects of Medicines, http://www.mhra.gov.uk/Safetyinformation/ Generalsafetyinformationandadvice/Adviceandinformationforconsumers/ Sideeffectsofmedicines/

for anything. Instead, you should consider social monitoring tools like Google Alerts and subscribing to specific online publications so that you receive their updates in your email inbox.

- Set a Google Alert[90] by visiting google.com/alerts and punching in your search term. Google will record this term, and each time new content appears in the newsfeed that contains the term, you will be notified via email. Set terms like "MS cure" and "multiple sclerosis research" to auto-pilot your search.
- Otherwise, visit blogs like sciencedaily.com and msif.org and subscribe to them. Each time they post new research, you will get it straight into your inbox. Then each morning or evening when you review your emails, you can glance to see if anything interesting has come up or not.
- Set a time each week to surf around the Net and look for any new research or cure potential. As you find new things, set alerts for them to follow their progress. This needs to be done every week so that your knowledge never outdates—but if you are a very busy person, then once a month will do.

You should also think about subscribing to big news platforms like nytimes.com and washingtonpost.com because they tend to have the latest news in their feeds long before anyone else does, which can be beneficial.

When you check in online, it would help to use the Google news tab instead of the general search area. It will give you a mixture of media instead of breaking news media, which is what you are interested in. Keep up with modern research to continue educating yourself on your options and to continue your recovery journey.

---

90   Matthew Woodward, The Ninja's Guide to Google Alerts, http://www.searchenginejournal.com/the-ninjas-guide-to-google-alerts/48068/

Gaining Family Support for MS Recovery

Depending on your family, it will be hard on them to accept your diagnosis and deal with all the changes going on around them because of it. Give them time and the opportunity to want to help before making any demands on them.

I believe that when an MS patient has a supportive family, keeping to specific eating and exercise routines is a lot easier. And this is the treatment that reduces your MS attacks, so you need to take this seriously. It will be so much harder for you if your spouse or kids—or parents—are not participating in your recovery.

Sit them down and explain what needs to change. The way that you live needs to change, and that includes how you eat, how you exercise, and how you de-stress. Invite them to do it with you, and educate them about the many health benefits of self-care in the modern age.

If you have kids already, there is a chance that one or more of them could one day end up being diagnosed with MS.[91] Getting them on a diet and exercise plan will help them maintain their health, and this will make the onset of the disease microscopic, or the disease may never take hold because of it.

Aside from that, there are numerous health benefits of eating a sugar-free, wheat- and gluten-free diet that thrives on nutrients from raw vegetables. Everyone will feel happier and healthier, and this will help keep the stress levels lower later on.

For now, you will have to see what they say. It can be difficult for family members, but support comes in all forms. If they cannot eat what you eat, then perhaps they can support you by driving you around when you cannot do it for yourself or be there for you emotionally. Families that stick together during these times get closer, and recovery is a faster process.

---

91   MS in Family Members, http://www.overcomingmultiplesclerosis.org/Recovery-Program/MS-in-Family-Members/

Nurturing a Culture of Self-Care

Your family will be living with you, and even if they do not partake in your new daily routines and eating schedules, they will be exposed to your renewed efforts to look after yourself. This means openly exploring how to relax more, eat healthier food, and exercise in a way that truly benefits your body.

When you become an advocate for self-care, your family will be able to see how much better life can be if they look after themselves properly. This will motivate them to eat healthier, exercise more often, and practice keeping stress at bay.

As an MS patient, you should think about nurturing a culture of self-care in your family. And this is because self-care inspires more of the same. When you look for healthier things to eat as a family, it becomes fun and a real adventure. When you do it alone, it can feel isolated and like no one cares what you are going through.

It is really hard to sit at a dinner table and eat protein with vegetables when across from you your entire family is eating a huge bowl of store-bought pasta. Your strength will come from your family, and they need to be committed for you.

If you cannot get them to support you by living your new lifestyle with you, then you should at least inspire them to be better and look after themselves with closer attention to detail. You only get one life, one body, and one chance to be healthy. You more than anyone know that it is only when your health is gone that you miss it.

Talking With Friends and Family About Your Needs

I believe that my busy lifestyle and highly stressed out state was what could have triggered my MS. It could be the reason your MS was triggered, too. That is why I want to bring the importance of practicing self-care to the fore and why you should stop placing the needs of others ahead of your own needs. You may need to change the way you live.

I was very much like that in my career. I worked constantly, always had somewhere to be and someone to assist, and barely ever stopped to do anything for myself. I ate erratically, I never considered the impact of all the work pressure, and I supported everyone through their hard times. It resulted in a disease that forced me to stop and think about myself.

Now that you have this disease and the threats that come with it (an attack could erupt at any time), you no longer have the option. Your needs must come first. This means openly communicating in a way that will help your friends and family understand that you have to dial back the support, effort, and engagement.

Remember that when you were diagnosed with MS, your family was also given the bad news. Their lives will change along with yours, but you need to make sure that this change is positive and does not harm your relationships by causing anger or resentment.

The Healing Power of Collaboration

At the same time, I want you to consider the dynamics involved in your personal MS medical team. There is a good chance that on your MS journey, you will have a family physician, a neurologist, a reflexologist, a dietician, an acupuncturist, a herbalist, and several other kinds of either medical or alternative staff on your team.

I do not see the benefit in keeping your conventional medicine doctors apart from your other healers. It makes far more sense for them to collaborate on making your MS symptoms vanish. When your neurologist is willing to read a report from your herbalist or acupuncturist, that is when real healing will begin.

I believe both sides of the medical field have good things to offer. Be discerning, and choose doctors that are open minded and willing to collaborate instead of compete. If you have this team of experts working on your case, it will supplement your own self-care regimen, and you will become an empowered patient.

This type of patient self-prescribes; they listen to their body, spirit, and mind; and they use intuition to guide them towards solutions.[92] I have personally experienced this process and come out the other side much, much healthier for it.

Your doctors need to collaborate for your good health. This is perhaps the most difficult element of self-care, but it is a huge bonus for you. It is sad that in this time of knowledge we are still forced to choose sides. If you can find an MS team to collaborate on making you well again, the chances are you will get there faster.

With advice from both sides of the field, you will be able to make educated decisions from a multitude of opinions that matter and are case specific. This will fuel your own personal investigations into what works for your body.

When to Visit the Doctor

MS can be light and irritating, and it can be severe and debilitating depending on the type that you have. Some symptoms, however, need to be immediately checked out by your doctor if they crop up, or additional damage could result.

That is why it is important that you visit the doctor when your vision has drastically changed and resulted in disability. Seriously blurred vision, double vision, or loss of vision coupled with other symptoms can leave you in need of help.

These symptoms can include coordination concerns, cognitive issues, dizziness, bladder trouble, and strange sensations in your body. After your diagnosis, if you relapse and any of these symptoms worsen, you will have to go to see the doctor.

---

92   Lissa Rankin, Collaboration Trumps Competition in Health Care, http://www.psychologytoday.com/blog/owning-pink/201201/collaboration-trumps-competition-in-health-care

You should also go if your attacks suddenly become more frequent or severe[93] and if a new symptom suddenly erupts that is causing you pain or distress. Your doctor is there to check your physical health, to run tests, and to determine what may have caused the new flare up.

This is a great time to take along your health and wellness journal, if you have been keeping one. It will be brimming with clues that you can narrow down to a fine art. Then if you want to relieve symptoms with alternative treatments, you should make regular appointments and include them in your routine.

I go for regular massages, which keeps my body loose and the blood flowing. It also helps reduce tension, which is a big one for me. You can do the same with your herbalist, acupuncturist, or reflexologist. They will help monitor your physical progress.

Alternative healthcare practitioners can be expensive because they are generally not covered by insurance and are payable out of pocket. Make sure that you take this into account when sourcing them.

---

93   Multiple Sclerosis (MS) – When to Call a Doctor, http://www.webmd.com/multiple-sclerosis/tc/multiple-sclerosis-ms-when-to-call-a-doctor

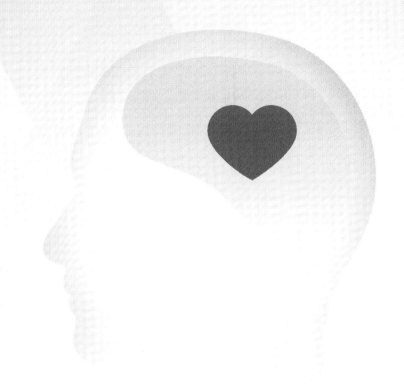

CHAPTER **11**

Managing Dangerous Stress Levels

"The truth is that stress doesn't come from your boss,
your kids, your spouse, traffic jams, health challenges,
or other circumstances. It comes from your thoughts
about these circumstances."

ANDREW BERNSTEIN

Stress is a silent killer and one that has managed to slip beneath the radar for patients with MS. But there are many experts that agree that stress may be a contributing activator for the disease. In fact, many studies have been conducted on how stress is related to multiple sclerosis, and it is even recognized as a trigger for attacks.

As someone with MS, you will need to learn to manage your stress levels so that they do not end up making your health worse. Dangerous stress levels cause a host of issues in the human body that you should be aware of and actively try to avoid.

Stress–Anxiety–MS Connection

Studies have proven that major life events can trigger MS attacks because of aggravated stress levels that affect your disease and general wellbeing. UCLA scientists[94] have shown through animal and human

---

94   Stress and MS, http://www.overcomingmultiplesclerosis.org/About-MS/Causes-of-MS/Stress/

study that MS relapses cause worsening disability and that these are directly related to stress, inflammation, and degeneration.

One third of all MS patients also struggle with serious anxiety—and because the disease is unpredictable and anything can set it off, this is a real concern for patients living with constant stress. Feeling anxious, worried, irritable, depressed, or low does not help when you are trying to remain positive about living with MS.

While stress is a normal part of life, leaving your body in a constant state of anxiety with raised cortisol levels is not. You need to find methods to control your stress before it triggers any additional damage.

Why Stress Will Be the End of You

A patient with MS can control their diet, their exercise routine, and the environment around them—but many will struggle to control their stress levels. There is a good chance that you were a stressed person before being diagnosed, and the diagnosis only sent you into fresh fits of stress that have made you even more bogged down with anxiety.

Having MS is stressful. For me, MS creates underlying worry, which is stressful and chronic. I wonder what is coming next, whether my symptoms will get worse, and if I will be able to handle my disease. It is not easy. Dr. David Mohr from the Behavioral Medicine Research Center[95] in California has conducted stress studies.

In these studies, a clear link between higher stress levels and the triggering of MS has been established. The conclusion of these studies was that stressful events worsen MS and should be avoided at all costs. If not, more severe impairment could be left behind from the attack, causing the patient to have to recover for longer periods and live with disability.

---

95   Daniel J DeNoon, Study: Stress Bad for MS, http://www.webmd.com/multiple-sclerosis/news/20040318/study-stress-bad-for-ms

Many more research studies have been conducted into the mind–body connection in multiple sclerosis. Dr. Quig, a clinical neuropsychologist at Georgetown University MS Center,[96] gave a revealing talk on stress, outlining how it is the unconscious response to "demand" that either helps or harms patients.

When you are under acute stress, your body releases hormones like adrenaline and cortisol, which raise your blood pressure, boost energy supplies, and increase your heart rate. When you have a nonessential fight or flight situation, this state becomes detrimental to your body over prolonged periods. This stress will constantly provoke your MS!

The Stress Flare-Up: Management Concerns

In order to prevent MS attacks or flare-ups, it then becomes critical to focus on managing your stress levels with greater purpose. Stress management is the art of keeping your body stress-free by releasing that stress in healthy ways and practicing control over your thoughts, emotions, and physical habits.

Eating right and getting enough exercise will already contribute to keeping your stress levels down. Some stress is good because it promotes learning, growth, and change. When this balance tips and stress becomes harmful, you will experience negative side effects from it.

- You need to come to terms with your disease and your new way of living. Yes, it is stressful having to manage a serious disease, but when that disease is greatly impacted by stress, you have to make the choice.

- Steer clear of stimulants like coffee, energy drinks, sugar, nicotine,[97] and other drugs, and get enough sleep. Lack of sleep

---

96   Lisa Emrich, Stress and MS: The Mind-Body Connection, http://www.healthcentral. com/multiple-sclerosis/c/19065/156041/stress/

97   Stress, http://www.msfocus.org/stress.aspx

is one of the leading hidden causes of stress as your body has to compensate for running "on empty."

- Emotional stress is the hardest one to fight. MS causes emotional distress that often leads to depression. You may want to consider going for therapy to deal with this new challenge or forming a supportive network of friends and family so that you always have someone to talk to about your disease.

Dr. Mohr's study later concluded that practicing stress management therapy[98] reduced the development of new brain lesions, which means that actively managing the way that you respond to demands helps to monitor and reduce MS attacks.

There is light at the end of the tunnel for you, however, as stress management comes with droves of other benefits for your body. In a naturally overstressed world, it pays to calm your body and your mind and vent that stress in healthy ways.

Practicing Meditation to Reduce Symptoms

Meditation may be foreign to you, but it is the quickest, cheapest method of reducing stress that is known in the world today. If you do not practice meditation, then you need to consider taking it up. If you do not know how to relax or truly unwind, the act of meditation can be the release you have been searching for.

Spend a few minutes meditating every day in the morning. Begin by folding your legs in a comfortable position. Close your eyes, and clear your mind. You can also use this opportunity to recite positive affirmation in your mind or to focus on positive thoughts. Allow all negative and distracting thoughts to trail away.

Practice breathing techniques that relax your body and lighten your stress levels. Inhale through your nose, and try to fill your belly

---

98   Jeri Burtchell, Study Shows That Stress Can Lead to MS Flare-Ups, http://www.healthline.com/health-news/ms-stress-could-predict-ms-disease-activity-121813

with air. Exhale through your mouth until you are breathing deeply and naturally. Research[99] has shown that meditation on a daily basis may alter your brain's neural pathways, which means that you will be more resilient to stress.

This deep breathing slows your heart rate, helps lower your blood pressure, and keeps your physical symptoms of stress under control. Regular meditation does in fact make you better equipped to handle stress because it allows your body to exist in a relaxed state for a while, free of concern and worry.

As you meditate, make sure that you are mentally present. Be aware of your body or of the way it feels on the ground. If you're new to meditation, work your way up to meditating for 25 minutes each day; make it consistent for best results. If you only meditate every now and then, you will not build up a stress resistance that will reduce your MS symptoms.

Taking Up a Calming Sport

Reducing stress is one of the top three techniques in reducing your chance of getting an MS attack that causes more symptoms. Physical activity has often been linked with stress reduction, and enjoying regular cardio exercise does wonders for that. But you can also combine stress reduction and activity in a calming sport.

The top two sports that come to mind are Tai Chi and yoga. Both are slow movement sports, but they focus on breathing, muscle tone, and being present—just like meditation does. Tai Chi was developed for self-defense, but it is so graceful that it promotes serenity through flowing movement.

The great thing is that even when you are not physically able to do a sport, you can still do Tai Chi because it is easy on the joints and muscles. You pick your pace and practice this art for 30 minutes a day for best results.

99   Jeannette Moninger, 10 Relaxation Techniques That Zap Stress Fast, http://www.webmd.com/balance/guide/blissing-out-10-relaxation-techniques-reduce-stress-spot

Yoga, on the other hand, is more mainstream, and it works. This calming sport uses breathing, meditation, controlled physical movement, and stretching to achieve its goals. Actively practicing yoga has been proven to reduce anxiety and stress, lower cortisol levels and blood pressure, improve sleep quality, and improve strength and muscle tone.[100]

Yoga and Tai Chi should become a part of your regular day. Both great for the mornings or just before you settle into bed for the night. There are also variations of these like Yogolates, which is Pilates combined with yoga.

Sport is always good for your health, but when stress management is high on your priority list, you need to take a more calming approach to your health.

Exploring the World of Positive Affirmations

Positive affirmations were once a part of junk science until they moved into the modern world with psychologists, coaches, and health practitioners. There is a lot of bad practice in the field, with people using positive affirmations to sell products instead of giving it the credibility that it deserves.

PLOS One published a study[101] stating that self-affirmations can protect against the damaging effects of stress on problem-solving performance—and this from researchers at Carnegie Mellon University. Clearly, there is something to be said about including positive affirmations in your average daily routine.

Defined, a positive affirmation is a statement that is meant to be repeated over time in order to boost the user's self-perspective or esteem. Something like "I am calm, stress-free, and living life

---

100 Elizabeth Scott, The Benefits of Yoga for Stress Management, http://stress.about.com/od/tensiontamers/p/profileyoga.htm

101 Ray Williams, Do Self-Affirmations Work? A Revisit, http://www.psychologytoday.com/blog/wired-success/201305/do-self-affirmations-work-revisit

healthily" is a good example of a positive affirmation. My personal favorite is "As you think so shall you be." They can be used in meditation, in yoga, and even in Tai Chi.

It is up to you to explore the world of positive affirmations. I have found them to be quite useful, as you can often get caught up in negative self-talk from the MS progression. It is important to remain positive, and this can be achieved through repetition. Say something enough and eventually you will begin to believe it.

There are many practical implications when using these affirmations to reduce stress. You can use them to motivate yourself to stick to your new diet or a new exercise routine or to simply get out there and be happier about your life. When a disease like MS crops up, suddenly everything is overshadowed by it.

It will help you to create a list of positive affirmations to reinforce any progress you have made and to use them repeatedly when you are exercising. You can also say them in front of the mirror every day when you are getting dressed.

Mindset and Overcoming MS

When you are first diagnosed with MS, an overwhelming fear and terror grip you. Then, each time you have to live through an attack, the fear comes back. That is the terrible thing about MS—you do not know when or how it will strike; you can only work to minimize the damage on every level: socially, emotionally, mentally, and physically.

A huge part of this is getting over the shock of diagnosis. You need to adjust your mindset now that you have so much more to do to remain healthy and mobile. You cannot afford to allow the disease to make you depressed and to neglect yourself even more. Self-care is vital to survival and growth, and you need to learn that early on.

There is real power in positive thinking. The resilience that you gain from it allows you to meet any challenge with optimism and focus. This branch of study[102] is known as positive psychology, and it has been changing lives since 1985, when a study was conducted on optimism and coping and later published in *Health Psychology*.

Every single day matters to you now, which means that you need to be positive as much as possible. With so many daily challenges, you cannot afford to be negative about your approach. When you change your mindset and begin choosing to see the positive in things, your brain will rewire itself to spot more positives in the world than negatives.

Of course it is all right to acknowledge your emotions—including anger, fear, and frustration. The key is in being aware of what you are feeling and then choosing a perspective or mindset that fully supports you. What are you creating? In doing so, you can quickly pick yourself up and focus on being more determined. There is no point mourning for a life you could have had; this is your only life! You have MS—now do the best you can with it. You can overcome it if you place your positive energy into doing just that.

How a Negative Mindset Causes Stress

A negative mindset is different from depression, but one often follows the other if left unchecked. Depression is the ugly MS accomplice that lurks in the shadows, waiting to grab you if you are having a bad day or a bad relapse. At all costs, you cannot allow a negative mindset to sneak in. Negative mindsets are usually what cause enough stress for you to eventually succumb to depression and then keep it going—taking you to dark places.

Negative thoughts are not reality. They are a pessimistic barrage of "what ifs" that can cause you so much stress that you have a relapse. We are all bound by our emotions, but large portions of the population cling to negative thoughts like the sky is falling on their

---

102 Lisa Emrich, MS and Positive Thinking, http://www.healthcentral.com/multiple-sclerosis/c/19065/153627/rewire/

heads. This Chicken Little tactic does nothing to reduce stress, aid recovery, and promote good health.

You could say that negative thoughts are a precursor to depression, just like positive thoughts are a precursor to happiness. Thoughts are a choice that you make and a habit that you form. You need to learn to let go of these negative thoughts, recover from them, and correct yourself when you begin to dwell on them too much.

A negative mind always sees the downside or "worst case scenario" in every situation.[103] But life does not play out like that. It is largely based on your decisions. For example, if you are having MS leg pain, you can choose to lie in bed and feel sorry for yourself, obsessing about the pain and complaining about your lack of mobility.

A positive person, however, would actively try to stop the pain by maintaining a routine that promotes health. They understand that even though their legs might hurt today, the quicker they can recover, the better off they will be, with less damage to their nerves. They will eat right, exercise as much as possible, and be cheerful in their approach.

The only difference between these two cases is stress. The negative person fears the worst instead of living for the best. You need to make this mindset switch to save yourself a lot of empty worry, stress, and useless depression.

A positive attitude has been my secret weapon against MS. It is what has guided me to seek healing and to believe that I can find ways to thrive in spite of my diagnosis. I strongly encourage you to begin nurturing one right away!

Relieving Stress: Five Methods

Stress arises when you lose control and can no longer cope with your circumstances. In the beginning with MS, this will happen a lot. It is

---

103 Erika Krull, Depression and Letting Go of Negative Thoughts, http://psychcentral.com/lib/depression-and-letting-go-of-negative-thoughts/0003764

also the reason why routines are so important to maintain because they promote a positive mindset by side-stepping worry. When you are actively working on your health, it is far easier to see the light.

- If you feel overwhelmed at work or at home, stop and take a moment. Meditation and breathing techniques can travel with you, and there are apps now that allow you to listen to calming music as you unwind. Even five minutes of this can defuse a mounting stress bomb. Practice it often.

- Laugh as often as you can. When you smile and laugh often, your stress will dissipate, and your body will reboot. Your brain is connected to your emotions and your physical body—even if you are not feeling happy, engaging in laughter quickly changes that when you need a release.

- Find social support.[104] MS is impossible to deal with alone; you need people you can talk to. Relieve stress by seeing a psychologist or by chatting about your disease with friends and family who are willing to help you in any way they can.

- Do a locational. In psychology, when stress is nipping at you, sometimes it helps to place both feet firmly on the ground and remind yourself where you are and that everything is going to be okay. Be present in your location, and remember that things often appear far worse than they are.

- Hypnosis can help to relive stress if you go in for professional sessions. In this state, you can be calmed and get that rest you need, even if it is for a little while. MS patients with large stress concerns should consider this weekly to improve their mental state and recover from depression or negative thinking.

Five Practical Strategies for Cortisol Reduction

104 Social Support: Tap This Tool to Beat Stress, http://www.mayoclinic.org/healthy-living/stress-management/in-depth/social-support/art-20044445

Cortisol is also called your body's "stress hormone" because it places your system on high alert in times of stress. While this is excellent if you are being attacked by a lion, it is horrible in your normal daily life. When your body is in a constant state of stress, it cannot recover and becomes prone to illness, fatigue, and additional side effects.

Keep your cortisol levels low to help manage your stress. To do this, pick any of these five strategies and practice them when you can.

- While meditating, tune in to different frequencies by saying "Om" like the Buddhists do. Studies from Maharishi University suggest that you can reduce cortisol by an additional 20%[105] simply by saying this word during meditation.

- Rid yourself of cortisol by getting enough sleep. Lack of sleep[106] forces the cortisol levels in your blood to remain elevated due to chronic sleep deprivation. Sleeping for six hours instead of eight may be doing this to you. Turn off the TV and the radio, and dim the lights—and get some sleep!

- Lose weight by eating a healthy diet. Another reason to lose weight is to prevent cortisol from storing fat in your body automatically, which it does. Lose weight, and it will become easier to regulate your levels.

- Put on your favorite calming music. Studies have shown that music alters the brain for the better when it is under enormous stress. Just listening to some music can reduce your stress response to pain and a host of other concerns.

- One of my go-to techniques is massage. When you go for regular massages, you can end up reducing your cortisol levels by one third. A good massage can increase dopamine and serotonin in your body that will make you feel better too.

---

105 Elizabeth Svoboda, 8 Ways to Beat Your Stress Hormone, http://www.prevention.com/mind-body/emotional-health/how-lower-cortisol-manage-stress

106 Want to Sleep Better? First, Reduce Your Cortisol Levels Then Follow These Six Key Steps, http://bodyecology.com/articles/reduce_your_cortisol_levels.php#.U9suAfmSySo

Practice keeping your cortisol levels low to control your stress and keep depression at bay. I have found these to be very useful when used in a regular routine for compounding benefits. Test which techniques you enjoy the most!

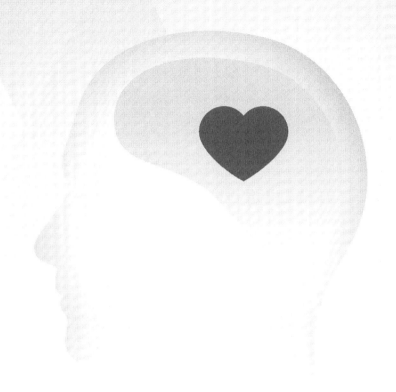

CHAPTER **12**

Exercise Your MS Away: Here's How

"I am only one, but still I am one. I cannot do everything, but still I can do something; and because I cannot do everything, I will not refuse to do something I can do."

EDWARD EVERETT HALE

Multiple sclerosis attacks the central nervous system, which means that pain is something you are going to be experiencing in different forms. From tingling, pain, and numbness to spasms, twitches, and weakness, exercising is a challenge.

The good news is that most of the time you should be symptom free, which means that you will have the energy, stamina, and physical capability to engage in exercise and keep your body healthy. But there are new rules that you need to acknowledge.

Can You Exercise With MS?

Yes, the simple answer is that you can exercise with MS. Exercise and human movement are critical to normal physical functioning, and the less you exercise, the more exposed your body will be to further dysfunction. If you want to improve mobility, then you need to do something to prevent the loss of muscle function and strength—even if it means seeing a physical therapist.

The difference is that when you have MS, you need to approach exercise[107] from a new perspective. That means identifying the types of exercise that will benefit you and the types that will not. This includes how long you should exercise for and how intense that workout should be. Under and over exercising are both big no-no's for you now.

Overheating is also a concern, as many MS patients are sensitive to heat. Taking cold showers can alleviate this, along with making sure that you are properly hydrated. If symptoms get worse during exercise, stop until you cool down.

No matter your age or physical limitations, you need to make sure that you exercise as often as possible; ideally, each day.

Why Many Modern Doctors Disagree

When a doctor assesses your physical status, they may restrict your exercise routine to make you more comfortable. Because many doctors do not get involved in diet and exercise as treatment for their patient's MS, this can sometimes come across as a warning against exercise as a whole, which is not the case.

If you tell a doctor that you are experiencing leg pain, for example, and cannot walk well, they are not going to motivate you to walk. If you suffer from serious fatigue, pain, and weakness, they may mention that exercise could make your symptoms worse.

While it is true that you should not push yourself and cause additional stress and damage, managing the way you exercise and the frequency of your exercise routine is key to recovering from MS. Relapsing and remitting MS will only stay away if routine is established, and this cannot happen if you are too afraid to exercise.

- If you exercise properly and listen to your body, you can exercise just as effectively as everyone else. Exercise does not

---

107 Multiple Sclerosis and Exercise, http://www.webmd.com/multiple-sclerosis/guide/multiple-sclerosis-exercise

make your MS symptoms worse or cause a relapse of previously aggregated symptoms.

- The right exercise will improve your mood, increase strength and mobility, decrease fatigue, prevent weight gain, improve sleep, improve your digestive system, and increase clarity in your thinking.

Many modern doctors may make you fearful of exercise, but you should never be afraid of it. You know what is going on inside your body, and you know what you can take. As long as you carefully restrict your exercise, it can only do your body good.

There have been lots of studies[108] that have confirmed that exercise for MS is very useful, but you should consult your doctor to check with them before beginning any new routine. This will ensure that you do not over or under exercise, backed up by expert opinion.

Proof That Exercise Improves Mental Function

A study conducted by the Center for Brain Health at the University of Dallas Texas,[109] has proven beyond doubt that exercise—specifically engaging in a regular exercise regimen—helps adults improve memory, brain function, and fitness. If you want to stay mentally sharp during your journey with MS, then exercise needs to be a critical part of it.

With a disease like MS, keeping your mental faculty is going to require hard work and dedication by selecting the right exercises for your body to work through every day. You do not need a performance-based exercise regimen, but it certainly helps if your daily exercise varies with cardio, weights, and sport-based exercise.

---

108 MS & Exercise, http://www.tysabri.com/ms-and-exercise.xml

109 Study Finds Aerobic Exercise Improves Memory, Brain Function and Physical Fitness, http://www.brainhealth.utdallas.edu/blog_page/study-finds-aerobic-exercise-improves-memory-brain-function-and-physical-fi

Many MS patients suffer from decreased cognitive ability that can impact speech, memory, and the way that they relate to other people. These challenges are among the most difficult to overcome, as sometimes they can be so severe you have to re-teach yourself how to do basic things after an MS attack.

Brain damage is not the most common symptom, but it happens. If you want to assist your body in warding off neurological dysfunction and cognitive impairment, then you need to seriously consider exercising for at least an hour every single day.

If your exercise is broken into light walks, yoga, and swimming, then great. Only you know what you can handle, but setting physical goals for yourself to overcome past damage is part of the process. I have seen people recover from serious debilitation simply by putting their minds to it and then sticking to a regular schedule. It makes all of the difference in the long term as long as you are getting enough nutrients for repair.

The Rest-Exercise Program Study

The rest-exercise method of getting fit and staying healthy is specifically for MS patients. It works by allowing you to move at your own pace and recover from any physical ailment while at the same time taking precautions to not overheat or trigger a stress response.

- People with MS usually show poor aerobic fitness even when the disease is caught early. If you have mild to moderate MS, however, you can recover your fitness levels if you dedicate yourself to 60 minutes a day of light aerobics. This will improve your aerobic fitness.

- Muscular fitness is also essential as your skeletal function is affected by MS. Reduced muscle power is a serious concern, especially for people in active fields.

- Pulmonary fitness is a key element because MS tends to decrease the strength of your ventilator muscles, which increases your risk of respiratory complications. Have your function assessed, and include exercises to recover.

- Immune function is the final frontier and will involve consistent and varied physical activity, so it helps to be involved in many different types of exercise.

Always warm up before you engage in physical activity[110] and then use the rest–exercise method to build stamina. Begin with 10-minute sessions at low intensity and work your way up to what feels comfortable. If you need to rest after 10 minutes, then rest. Then continue once you have cooled down and rejuvenated.

Do not forget to stretch and stay cool, and focus most of your attention on cardio exercise. Train in bursts like this to take stock of how you feel afterwards. If you cannot do any more , always stop. Do what you can; no more, no less.

Working With Cardio and MS

With cardio, you can start slowly, which makes it an ideal beginner exercise for MS patients that have suffered recent relapses. MS research widely supports cardio exercise because it improves symptoms of fatigue and your overall quality of life.

If you raise your heart rate regularly, it decreases the progression of the disease and results in fewer brain lesions and atrophy. This is enough to get any MS patient on a treadmill or running down the road! Cardio has huge MS benefits, so make it a habit of yours.

While it is true that cardio–respiratory fitness[111] reduces your exercise tolerance, researchers have found that you will experience more benefits than the average person from exercising because it has the potential to do so much good in your body.

---

110 Multiple Sclerosis and Exercise, http://www.webmd.com/multiple-sclerosis/guide/multiple-sclerosis-exercise

111 Joanna Kileff, Aerobic Exercise for People With Multiple Sclerosis, http://www.mstrust.org.uk/professionals/information/wayahead/articles/08022004_03.jsp

In the past, doctors would tell MS patients to "take it easy," and their exercise regimens would vanish, contributing to their degeneration. Cardio is great for flexibility as well, and it wards off muscle shortening and weakness. Patients with severe spasticity should spend time stretching before cardio for at least 20 minutes to an hour.

In addition, it is up to you how you choose to spend your cardio time. Bike rides, running, hiking, or any other incredible cardio sports are all available to you. I strongly suggest, however, investing in a treadmill for your home so that you can guarantee walks or runs during your average day.

That way if you have a relapse, you will not have any excuses and will have a method of exercising, even if it is mild.

Working With Weights and MS

A balanced exercise routine[112] always involves resistance training with weights or some other form of resistance. Your muscles will need all of the help they can get to recover from inactivity after a relapse, so resistance training can improve muscle strength, coordination, efficiency, functional ability, and energy levels.

Weight training does not trigger MS unless it makes you incredibly stressed out. A properly executed training program will not cause additional fatigue or distress unless you overheat. That is why it is important that you watch how hot you get.

In the beginning, you may experience muscle soreness and a temporary worsening of their symptoms. But ultimately, your body improves over time. You should focus on resistance training at least twice a week, especially if you have unstable blood pressure or heart concerns that limit your cardio function.

---

112 Strength Training and Multiple Sclerosis, http://www.msaustralia.org.au/sites/default/files/Strength%20training%20and%20multiple%20sclerosis%20-%20Updated%20Aug%2011.pdf

My advice would be to approach a sports scientist or speak to your doctor about helping you create a weight training regimen that you can manage effectively at your current stage of disability. If you have a relapse, you will have to start building your strength and stamina from the beginning again.

Keep in mind that the healthier your muscles are, the better your mobility will be after relapses. This is the main reason to include strength and resistance training in your weekly exercise routine. It pays off when your health suffers.

Exploring "Other Activities" With MS

Just because you have MS does not mean that you have to stop enjoying any type of activity. I strongly advise you to start some sort of activity. Activities encourage ranges of motion that your body usually would not perform, and this is good for balance, coordination, muscle strength, and cardio.

Spend some time exploring other activities, such as Tai Chi or yoga, and find one that challenges you physically but is also fun and dynamic. Doing such activities on the weekends will give you some respite from your other exercise routines and the chance to socialize with people.

Before any activity is chosen, you need to sit down with your doctor and assess your disability level. The good news is that you can supplement your sporting routine with your other exercise routines and your stress management program, which may include Tai Chi and yoga. Physically speaking, there are some yoga teachers that are more fit than football players, so it is not a matter of choosing a less effective sport.

Exercising in the Cold: Swimming

Swimming is an excellent type of cardio workout for patients with MS because as you are exerting yourself, the water keeps you cool.

It becomes almost impossible to overheat when you are surrounded by water.

Plus, it gives you the opportunity to socialize, relax, and play. Few other sports have this mainstream appeal in a non-competitive environment. Strength training can also be easier in a swimming pool as the motion of kicking your legs and swinging your arms improves muscle tone and flexibility. I love to go to the pool and do resistance-training exercises with my coach. I use paddles and water weights to do upper-body exercises that get my heart rate up and use the pool steps to strengthen my leg muscles.

Because high levels of stress are associated with MS, swimming is a good way to combat this as it can be very relaxing. Few things are as peaceful as floating in a pool during those rest periods. So when you exercise in a pool, you get to exert yourself and rest in an ideal environment. I highly recommend exercising in a cold swimming pool.

Balance and coordination trouble can be improved through swimming, which are additional benefits for active MS patients that want to restore previous function. With the help of a coach, you can get into a swimming pool and exercise even if you have trouble balancing and walking on the ground.

This is called water or aqua therapy,[113] and it is why swimming is the go-to sport for MS patients that have suffered severe relapses. Swimming often speeds along the recovery in conjunction with nutrition and a positive mindset.

The MS Workout: Planning Your Schedule

Experimentation[114] is important when looking for an exercise schedule that works for you and your specific type of MS. Do not get

---

113 Ann Pietrangelo, Open Swim: Multiple Sclerosis Water Therapy, http://www.healthline.com/health/multiple-water-therapy

114 Exercising With Multiple Sclerosis, http://www.activemsers.org/exercisesstretches/tipsexercisingwithms.html

bogged down by what other people do. If you are uncertain of what type of exercise to do, then seek the professional advice of a therapist to avoid injury. A good balance would incorporate resistance training and cardio.

- Start with what you can manage. Do not be Superman! Begin by setting a time limit for yourself.
- You can also choose to exercise in increments—for 15 minutes in the morning, then 15 at lunchtime, then 15 at dinner—or something similar to this. By breaking up your exercise, you lower the risks of triggering an attack or overheating.
- Always take at least 15 minutes of warm ups into account. Find and perform range of motion exercises every single day to stay loose and to prevent shortening and shrinkage of your muscles. This will ward off the severity of your spasticity symptoms if you have any. Ideally, stretch before all exercise.
- It can be nice to focus on cardio one day, then swimming on another, and weights on an alternate day and so forth. This way you give your body time to recover after each bout, and you will not get bored with repetitive exercises that you cannot stick to.

In a similar way to testing your body with food, you need to test your body with exercise. Knowing what you enjoy and what hurts is only part of the solution. It needs to fit into your schedule because exercise has just become an important part of your life.

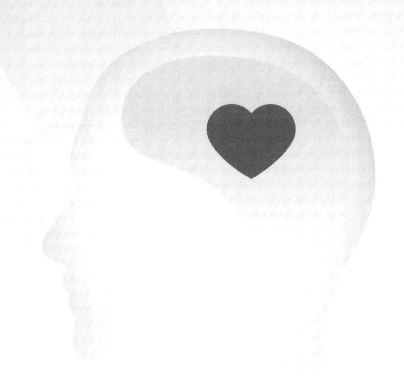

CHAPTER **13**

Working With Natural Supplementation

"By the proper intake of vitamins and other nutrients and by following a few other healthful practices from youth or middle age on, you can, I believe, extend your life and years of well-being by twenty-five or even thirty-five years."

LINUS PAULING

Natural supplements were once something that only gym junkies and super healthy people added to their diet for performance in sports and overall good health. But these days, being without supplements does more harm than good.

For people like us with MS, it becomes even more important to take natural supplements. Even the best modern diet can be lacking in nutrients, but when you take cooking and modern convection methods into account, what you are eating is not enough.

The Quality of the American Food Supply

Every time you eat, your body converts that food into the cells that will repair, heal, and make up your new systems. The saying "you are what you eat" is literally correct. The only problem with this is that when people switch from junk foods to fresh foods, they face a new, hidden threat—the dwindling nutrient supply in our current food sources.

The fact is that decades ago, food was much richer in vitamins, minerals, and trace elements than it is now. With the rising trends in soil depletion—combined with modern agriculture practice—soil just does not contain as many essential nutrients anymore.

When a farmer plants a pest-resistant crop that grows ultra-quickly, with each successive generation, the food source is less good for you than the previous one. New crops cannot absorb the nutrients that older crops once did, because they are made for commercial sale (growth rate and size) and not health (nutrient content).

The Kushi Institute[115] discovered in a study that compared nutrient data from 1975 to 1997 that 12 vegetables have a 27% reduced calcium count, 37% reduced iron count, 30% vitamin C count, and 21% vitamin A count. The latest studies are even worse than this, and because we have lost close to half of our nutrient supply, your body only gets half the nutrients.

Natural Healing: Herbs and Spices

Because of the shortage of nutrients in commercially grown food and the cooking methods that further diminish the nutrient content (frying, for example), you should be actively adding healing herbs and spices to your diet. These natural supplements promote good health and will help you physically recover from an MS attack.

In Chinese herbal medicine, they believe that multiple sclerosis symptoms can be effectively controlled using blends of herbs and spices. These theories have some weight, with a large study conducted by the Department of Neurology and Traditional Chinese Medicine in Fujian.[116] The results were impressive decoctions that were given to patients with great success. A decoction is the action or process of

---

115 Dirt Poor: Have Fruits and Vegetables Become Less Nutritious?, http://www.scientificamerican.com/article/soil-depletion-and-nutrition-loss/

116 Subhuti Dharmananda, Chinese Herbal Treatment for Multiple Sclerosis, http://www.itmonline.org/arts/msalsmg.htm

extracting the essence of something. In this instance, the herbs and spices were concentrated into an essence by heating or boiling and then were administered to patients.

Thirty-five patients were treated; three dropped out in the first 10 days, and some improvement was found. Two cases of MS were deemed "cured" after taking 45 of the 68 doses, 15 were markedly improved, and 15 were somewhat improved with 20–40 doses.

In Western medicine, many herbals and herbal supplements will help resort your health when your MS flares up. Cinnamon, for example, has lots of antioxidants, which is great for cognitive repair. Sage is excellent for stress and cognitive improvement, and turmeric (another great antioxidant) fends off plaque development and improves immune function.

MS patients should consider drinking chamomile tea to keep stress levels down and take the edge off. This acts as a mild muscle relaxant and can also have an anti-spasmodic effect. Chamomile is also great for facilitating quality sleep and better digestive health, which you could use.

Other types of herbs that can help in your recovery are green tea for an antioxidant boost; flaxseed and evening primrose herbs, which are good for essential fatty acids to reduce inflammation; and of course, the controversial herb that is still being legalized, medical marijuana.

Vitamins and Supplements: Do They Work?

There are huge volumes of evidence that prove vitamins and supplements are useful for people with autoimmune diseases like MS. Vitamin D, for example, is an essential vitamin for MS patients as it was discovered that MS is most prevalent in places where there is little sun, and therefore a shortage of natural vitamin D[117] occurs in sufferers.

---

117 Rebecca Oshiro, How Does Vitamin D Work in Multiple Sclerosis?, https://www. vitamindcouncil.org/blog/how-does-vitamin-d-work-in-multiple-sclerosis/#

Cells throughout your brain and spinal cord have vitamin D receptors. In studies where high doses of vitamin D were given to MS patients, their nerve damage was reduced. I recommend going on a vitamin D supplement as soon as possible if you are deficient, or spend more time out in the sun to soak up the positive benefits.

A daily multivitamin is also essential if you want to cover a broad range of potential deficiencies. Supplementation by adding powered vitamins and minerals to your morning juices can be handy and will facilitate uptake and regeneration in your body.

Keep in mind that natural supplements also have contraindications, which means that if they cause a reaction or make you feel worse, stop using them or adjust your dosage. Always keep your MS team and neurologist informed about the vitamins that you want to take so that they can give you advice to add to what you already know.

It is possible to eat lots more fresh foods, but they may be challenging to prep based on your daily schedule. Eating healthy foods and supplementing is the new modern way of becoming healthy again. What your food lacks, your supplements will make up for. You will need to test different supplements and see how they work for you. This is the best way to settle on specific brands.

Vitamins to Support MS Recovery

Here is an essential list of vitamins that you can use to support and facilitate your MS recovery. Adding these to your routine will only contribute to your health and wellness and may even prevent and protect against future MS attacks. Be cautious of vitamins that claim to boost your immune system[118] as they could contain stimulants and other undesirables.

The vitamins that you will want to focus on the most are called "antioxidant" vitamins because they promote the suppression of free radicals in your body.

---

118 Vitamins, Minerals and Supplements, http://multiplesclerosis.net/natural-remedies/vitamins-supplements/

- Vitamin A, or beta-carotene, is a good antioxidant for your eyes, especially if you have been having MS-related vision problems.

- Vitamin C and E (in combination with selenium) were proven to be well tolerated in a small MS study, and this combination tends to reduce the incidence of urinary tract infections, which are common in MS. Cranberries are a ready source of vitamin C if you do not want to take a supplement because of overdose concerns.

- Zinc is used in a lot of important functions in the body. People with MS tend to have low zinc levels, but there are studies that argue the opposite. In this case, if you have not gone for your dietician's analysis and had a full nutritional workup, you will not know if your levels are fine or not. If you lack zinc, supplement it.

- Vitamin K2 has traditionally been dismissed as a vitamin group that only works for blood clotting; however, K2 protects your body from heart disease; facilitates healthy skin, strong bones, and normal brain function; and supports growth and development—even reducing cancer prevalence.[119]

Your body needs these vitamins to maintain good health. Any deficiency could aggravate your MS symptoms and lead to great damage in the body. Once I had corrected my nutrient levels, I felt so much better. If your body is a machine and you do not give it the right oil, eventually it will rust, break, or stop working properly. Supplements are like adding high performance oil to the machine.

Other Supplements to Support MS Recovery

Along with the vitamins that you can choose to add to your daily diet, there are a number of health-promoting supplements that do

---

119 Chris Kresser, Vitamin K2: The Missing Nutrient, http://chriskresser.com/vitamin-k2-the-missing-nutrient

not fall into the vitamin category. These supplements can be the most beneficial of all, so you should talk to your doctors about them.

- GLA, or Gamma-Linoleic Acid,[120] is a great Omega 6 supplement, and studies suggest that it reduces inflammation in animal models with MS.
- Coenzyme Q10 is a classic and a particularly strong antioxidant used to improve your mitochondrial health. Decreased levels of this antioxidant have been responsible for many disease states, and it improves cognitive function.
- Selenium makes up for an MS patient's low levels of glutathione peroxidase, which is a powerful antioxidant. Adding more antioxidant-producing supplements can do incredible things for an MS patient.
- Lipoic acid is equally as beneficial as it passes the blood–brain barrier and decreases the activity of intercellular adhesion molecules, which play a role in the pathogenesis of MS. Experts believe that these molecules are responsible for allowing pro-inflammatory cells into your central nervous system.
- A recent study found that turmeric[121] helps fight MS as it blocks MS progression. It has been discovered that curcumin is remarkably anti-carcinogenic and anti-inflammatory and is brimming with antioxidants. It is a neuro-protectant that you want in your diet.
- Omega 3 Fatty Acids[122] are excellent supplements as they support brain health and neuro connection. The supplements

---

120   Health Concerns, http://www.lef.org/protocols/neurological/multiple_sclerosis_02.htm

121   Turmeric May Fight Multiple Sclerosis, http://www.whfoods.com/genpage. php?tname=news&dbid=43

122   Ronald Watson, Do Omega-3 Fatty Acids, Vital For Health and Therapy of Many Neurological Diseases, Modulate Multiple Sclerosis?, http://scitechconnect.elsevier.com/ omega-3-fatty-acids-vital-health-therapy-many-neurological-diseases-modulate-multiple-sclerosis/#.U_R4dPmSySo

help improve cognitive ability, and they reduce inflammation, which can prevent relapses.

- Medical marijuana, or cannabis,[123] has been found to significantly improve pain, ataxia, sleep disorders, spasticity, and anxiety in MS patients. Speak to your doctor about including it in your recovery plan if modern medicines become too much for you and you need something with fewer side effects.

- Glucosamine is extracted from shellfish shells and has been proven to suppress the animal form of MS in laboratory tests. This can be used alone or in conjunction with disease-modifying drugs.

If you are going to use more than one supplement, it is important that you talk to a doctor or dietician or herbalist about it beforehand as certain supplements can deactivate or change others. As in modern medicine, supplements and vitamins are not "safe at any dose," so please pay attention to how much you take.

Nutrient Boosts and Juicing

Nutritional therapy is a valid method of treating your MS. Juicing is one method of applying this therapy in the comfort of your own home. When you juice, it gives you the benefit of extracting all of the nutrients out of raw vegetables and fruit without having to eat and digest all of the fiber in these foods.

You might remember Dr. Wahls[124] and how she cured her MS with nutrients. She chalked up her MS to DNA, infections, toxin exposures, micronutrient intake, hormonal balance, food allergies,

---

123 Multiple Sclerosis Symptom Treatment With Medical Marijuana, http://www.medicalmarijuana.net/uses-and-treatments/multiple-sclerosis/

124 Dr Wahls' Super-Nutrient Paleo Diet, That Reversed Her Multiple Sclerosis, http://paleozonenutrition.com/2012/02/08/a-new-experiment-dr-wahls-super-nutrient-paleo-diet-9-cups-veggies-a-day/

and stress levels. Eventually she discovered that mitochondria need to function correctly in order for MS patients to recover.

She applied her theories and corrected her MS with food nutrients, eating up to nine cups of fresh vegetables daily and using juicing to deliver a lot of the nutrient goodness to her system. You can do the same thing by buying a juicer and having fun with the family by learning all about juice recipes.

I juice every single morning, and it makes me feel great. Add a little creative flavor, and you get to enjoy a nutrient-rich drink that has far-reaching health benefits for you.

Consider improving your nutrient profile by becoming a juicer. It was one of the best things I ever did, and it helped transform my health. I firmly believe that juicing will do the same for you if you spend the time needed to find delicious combinations of flavor. Check out Reboot With Joe to learn how to juice correctly: http://www.rebootwithjoe.com/category/blog/recipes/juice.

Vitamin D and Sunlight Exposure

According to the latest study by JAMA Neurology,[125] vitamin D was found to slow the progression of MS and even reduced harmful brain activity. The debate in the medical community rages on as many doctors refuse to prescribe vitamin D to their patients because there are no proven studies showing what D does to the immune system.

Doses of vitamin D are also tricky to get right because each MS patient is different. That said, Harvard professor Dr. Alberto Ascherio believes that vitamin D can be a huge benefit to MS patients. The study at JAMA proved that people with lower vitamin D levels get more brain lesions and have worsening symptoms than those with higher levels.

---

125 Steven Reinberg, Vitamin D May Slow Multiple Sclerosis: Study, http://www.webmd.com/multiple-sclerosis/news/20140120/vitamin-d-may-slow-multiple-sclerosis-study-suggests

This is why I advocate for vitamin D. Because while it is still being studied, there are growing bodies of evidence that prove it is important to autoimmune diseases. Infrequent outdoor activities and the use of sunscreen have been found to be risk factors in the development of MS because they block the absorption of vitamin D.[126]

In the study that proved this, people were most likely to be at increased risk in Norway between the ages of 13 and 18, while people aged 5 were at high risk in Italy. Parents should inform their kids that they should either be in the sun for short amounts of time or stay in the shade to get the vitamin D that they need.

Putting sunblock on prevents your body from absorbing the sun, and you need this if you are going to get your daily vitamin D. Otherwise, you will need to take a supplement, so make sure that it is a bioactive form of D and that you get your initial doses right. Popping two vitamin D tablets is preferable to leaving your levels low.

Getting In Your B Vitamin Range

With MS, you need your B vitamin range more than any other type of vitamin because of the constant fatigue that is so common in so many MS patients. Many people with MS do not realize that they have a B12 deficiency, but many do.

Having low levels of B12 in your body also makes your symptoms worse, so it makes sense to get on a B vitamin complex as quickly as possible. If the deficiency is low enough, doctors have found it to mimic MS in the body as it causes brain damage[127] and destruction of the myelin sheath and underlying axon.

---

126 New Study Shows Relationship Between Sun Exposure and Multiple Sclerosis in Norway and Italy, https://www.vitamindcouncil.org/vitamin-d-news/new-study-shows-relationship-between-sun-exposure-and-multiple-sclerosis-in-norway-and-italy/

127 Julie Stachowiak, Vitamin B12 and Multiple Sclerosis, http://ms.about.com/od/livingwellwithms/a/vitamin_b12.htm

As someone with MS, you will benefit from B12 in that it helps to maintain your myelin sheath because it plays a crucial role in the metabolism of fatty acids essential for the maintenance of myelin. Steroids have been found to reduce Bs in the body, which can be problematic if you are taking a steroid to treat your MS.

I suggest getting tested by your doctor for B12 along with doing your complete nutritional profile. Vitamin B6 is a natural energy booster, but it is also the one that causes tingling, numbness, or pain if taken in large doses. This is why it is best to buy a B12 vitamin and then a B6 separately to keep the dose low.

Getting your B vitamin range right will help you feel more energetic, and it will give your body the fuel it needs to repair your myelin after an MS attack. This is excellent knowledge to use if you are trying to recover from your last episode.

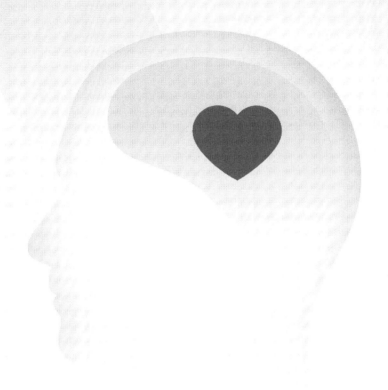

CHAPTER **14**

How Others Cope With MS

"Multiple Sclerosis is obviously close to my heart and I'm determined to make a difference in the lives of people who suffer from the disease by raising the profile of MS, as well as raising funds for advocacy and research."

ANN ROMNEY

Thanks to the Internet and the spread of news, it is easy to find out how other people have been dealing with their multiple sclerosis symptoms—especially celebrities and people in positions of power who have access to the best doctors in the world.

These folks can teach you a lot about overcoming struggle, looking after yourself, and living for today. These are their inspiring stories.

Montel Williams: Diet, Exercise, and Marijuana

Montel Williams is one of America's favorite television hosts and one of the most outspoken celebrities advocating for MS research today. He has even launched a new show, *Living Well With Montel,* to speak more about natural health and wellness.

After being diagnosed with multiple sclerosis in 1999, Montel's life changed. He graduated from the Naval Academy in 1980 and was on his way to get pre-commissioning inoculations when he lost 80% of his vision in his left eye.

He saw doctors from the Naval Academy and several other hospitals, but none could tell him why he had lost his vision. Montel was 22, in great shape, and an African American—almost the opposite of the Caucasian female MS stereotype. Because of this, it took him 19 years to be diagnosed after living with remitting and relapsing MS all that time.

Montel's MS affects his lower extremities, mainly with neuralgic pain from his knees to his feet on both sides. At one point the pain was so great that he attempted suicide. Since being diagnosed, Montel has taken every medication under the sun, with massive side effects.

The medication ruined his digestive system, and things got worse. Then he turned to natural remedies, even advocating publically for medical marijuana, which he says has reduced his consistent pain by 20–40% and his night tremors by 60%.[128]

Before going to bed every evening, Montel will use edible marijuana to control his pain, and he lives without medication—only a healthy, nutritious diet and regular exercise. Today, he continues to try to get medical marijuana legalized for MS patients in America.

His argument is that if a doctor can prescribe a patient morphine, which is massively damaging to the body, the same doctor should be able to prescribe medical marijuana—which works better than pain medication, with no negative side effects.

Jack Osbourne: Ketogenic Diet and Alternative Therapy

Jack Osbourne, son of the infamous rocker Ozzy Osbourne, was diagnosed with MS at the age of 26. His daughter was only a few weeks old when he began to experience problems with his vision. When he visited the doctor, he had lost 80% of his vision in his right eye.

---

128 Multiple Sclerosis: Montel Williams and MS, http://www.medicinenet.com/script/main/art.asp?articlekey=53785&page=2

The celebrity had starred in the popular show *The Osbournes* and *Jack Osbourne: Adrenaline Junkie*. He had become busy with work on producing and directing and was just starting his family like so many other newly diagnosed MS patients.

"MS is like a fingerprint because it affects everyone so differently," he revealed in an interview.[129] Jack controls his MS with medication and nutritional lifestyle changes. He still exercises regularly and is investigating holistic treatment options for the future.

The decision to use the Paleo low carb diet to treat the symptoms of multiple sclerosis has support by Dr. Terry Wahls, author of *The Wahls Protocol: How I Beat Progressive MS Using Paleo Principles and Functional Medicine*. In an exclusive interview, he explains how Dr. Wahls told him how she uses the high–fat, low-carb ketogenic diet combined with Paleo diet principles to treat herself and to help others with neurological conditions.[130]

Ann Romney: Equine Therapy, Alternative Treatment, and Diet

Ann Romney is the wife of Mitt Romney, the Republican nominee for the 2012 presidential election. She became first lady of Massachusetts when her husband became governor.

Ann was diagnosed in 1998 with relapsing and remitting MS—the most common kind. As a naturally athletic woman, the first symptoms to appear were stumbling, weak legs, and shaky hands. Because of her love for jogging, tennis, and skiing, she approached her brother, a doctor, who told her to see a neurologist.

---

129 Jack Osborne's Life-Changing Diagnosis, http://www.doctoroz.com/episode/jack-osbournes-life-changing-diagnosis

130 Jack Osbourne: High fat low-carb ketogenic Paleo diet helps multiple sclerosis. http://www.examiner.com/article/jack-osbourne-high-fat-low-carb-ketogenic-paleo-diet-helps-multiple-sclerosis

When she did go for an MRI, they spotted the lesions and diagnosed her with MS. She was given steroids to reduce the attacks, and they worked. But as is often the case, the side effects became too much to bear. She needed to be mobile and to recover.

Ann suffered from severe fatigue, so she took up equine therapy. The movements of a horse mimic natural human movement, enhancing strength, muscle flexibility, and balance. Slowly, her coordination returned, but her legs were still numb and weak. She used reflexology and acupuncture to help recover from her weakness.

Today she recommends that people find others with MS to draw personal strength from them. She did not do it in the beginning, but she found the right groups have merit. She is no longer on any form of modern medication and instead is using diet and alternative therapies to keep her healthy and in remission.

Even though this sometimes results in the occasional flare-up, Ann is doing much better than when she was first diagnosed. She also follows a careful eating plan and keeps exercising so that she can remain fit and mobile. These flare-ups can last from a few days to a few months depending on the severity, but she remains positive about it.

Trevor Bayne: Diet, Exercise, and Stress Management

Trevor Bayne is one of NASCAR's most popular drivers—winning the American NASCAR Spring Cup Series and Nationwide Series for racing. Like many other young people diagnosed with the disease, Trevor is in the best shape in his life.

At 22, he was faced with scrutiny as to the safety of his driving now that he had to live with MS, which causes loss of coordination—a skill essential to race car drivers. Doctors now clear him to race by physically assessing him before entry. He first noticed numbness in his arm during a race in Texas in 2011.

Originally, he thought the symptoms were related to an insect bite, but when they returned, he knew that he should have it checked out.

Some three weeks later, Trevor was admitted to the Mayo Clinic with fatigue, double vision, and nausea. They ruled out Lyme disease, and he began to go for regular check-ups as the symptoms progressed. Many of his friends and family say that he is fortunate to have received his diagnosis, as it would not have happened if he was not a famous race car driver.

Bayne completed his first triathlon in December[131] and does not take any medication at all for his MS. Instead, he focuses on eating properly and exercising in the right way, which helps to keep him symptom-free.

As a devout Christian, Trevor often gives motivational speeches to encourage others with MS to lead full and healthy lives. Even though he has a serious disease, he does not let it define him and continues living life in the fast lane.

Now he continues to race—and is extra careful about being checked out and given a clean bill of health before each race.

Richard Cohen: Positive Thinking and Clinical Trials

Richard Cohen is an award-winning journalist and author and was diagnosed with MS at the tender age of 25. As in many families, Richard's father and grandfather both had MS as well. He has lived with MS his entire life, and now, at the age of 66, he does his best with it.

Legally blind, Richard uses a cane and a wheelchair to get around. He has spoken publically on many occasions about how difficult losing his independence from this disease was. Now Richard has

---

131 Jacque Wilson, NASCAR Driver Trevor Bayne Diagnosed With Multiple Sclerosis, http://www.cnn.com/2013/11/12/health/trevor-bayne-multiple-sclerosis/

secondary progressive MS, which has taken its physical toll.

For this reason, he has offered himself to a new clinical trial using stem cells. He has hope that the stem cell therapy will help repair his damaged nervous system. A short while ago, a swollen foot landed him in the hospital, where a blood clot nearly reached his heart.

These days Richard is still positive about recovery, although after living with MS for 40 years, he dares not consider it. With trouble walking, a weak right side, and blindness, MS has done a lot to remove his independence from him.

He has never felt like a victim, even though back in 1973 all the medical establishment could do was prescribe harsh medications that caused additional damage to his body. He has written books about his struggle, namely, *Blindsided: Lifting a Life Above Illness*,[132] and how he manages the daily pain that he is forced to live with.

His story is enormously inspiring because he has never allowed MS or the debilitating effects to stand in his way. He worked all his life, became a hugely successful writer, and had a family with the woman he loved and is still married to. Inspiring!

Clay Walker: Diet, Exercise, and Stress Management

Clay Walker was one of the best country singers in the U.S. when he received his MS diagnosis back in 1996. Doctors told him that he would be in a wheelchair in four years and dead in eight. The prognosis was not great, but Clay could not accept that this was his fate.

It has been 18 years now since that gloomy prognosis. Thanks to his wife, Jessica, he has managed to stay on top of his disease and has helped manage his symptoms for many years. She makes sure that he exercises and eats nutritious food.

---

132 Richard Cohen on Why His Multiple Sclerosis Diagnosis Didn't Make Him a Victim, http://www.huffingtonpost.com/2014/01/20/richard-cohen-multiple-sclerosis_n_4632001. html

Early in Clay's career, his body gave him reminders that something was not right. He was a country music star, a recording artist, entertainer, husband, and father—things were hectic.

He first experienced tingling and numbness on his right side with facial spasms. They did not go away, so he went for tests. That was when he found out he had relapsing remitting MS at the age of 26.

Clay Walker manages his MS through routine exercise, healthy dieting, and taking his medication every day. He has also established a charity for people with MS, where he shares insight on how to manage the disease and contributes to finding the cure.

His charity is funded by Teva Pharmaceuticals,[133] and this allows him to reach out and educate people about the disease. His "Stick With It" campaigns have advocated for sticking with a solid regular routine for long-term health and wellness.

Clay has dealt with leg numbness, spasms, and serious coordination concerns that have made performing live a challenge. But he does it all with the support and love of his wife and family and, of course, his fans.

Tamia Hill: Medication and Diet

Tamia Hill is a famous R&B singer discovered by Quincy Jones in 1994. At 19 years old, she started recording and was quickly nominated for a Grammy Award. Some of her more famous works include collaborations with Brandy, Gladys Knight, and Chaka Khan.

Tamia released several albums between 1998 and 2003—then she was diagnosed with MS. She first started noticing symptoms when her husband, Grant, a professional basketball player, sustained a knee injury. While he recovered at home, she felt more tired than normal.

---

133 Mari Cartel, How Clay Walker Manages Symptoms of Multiple Sclerosis, http://www.lifescript.com/health/centers/multiple_sclerosis/articles/how_clay_walker_manages_symptoms_of_multiple_sclerosis.aspx

After that, she experienced numbness in her legs and in other parts of her body. They told her it was a pinched nerve, and she was sent home only to return a few weeks later. Things degenerated quickly, and she could barely move.

Finally, after long bouts of testing, she was diagnosed with MS. Despite the lack of a cure, she refuses to give in to the disease and stop performing. She takes injections every other day and eats right to manage the symptoms.

Tamia was better able to control her symptoms when she got pregnant[134] and her MS went into remission. She constantly reaches out to people experiencing strange symptoms and urges them to visit multiple doctors until they are satisfied with their diagnosis and treatment plan. If something does not feel right, it is not right she says.

After her own back-and-forth experience with doctors, she sympathizes with MS patients that are diagnosed late. The earlier you are diagnosed, the easier it becomes to learn how to manage your unique symptoms. Find the right roads as soon as you can to recover—and you can lead a perfectly normal and exciting life.

David Lander: Exercise, Diet, and Medication

David Lander, better known as Andrew "Squiggy" Squiggman from the popular television show *Laverne & Shirley* from 1976 to 1982, was diagnosed with MS in 1984. He often speaks about how he realized something was wrong—his legs would fall asleep, and he would get a tingly sensation in his fingers.

It went away and returned again one day, but this time it made walking down stairs difficult. He thought it was vertigo but later found out it was MS. After using Avonex, an MS medication, he

---

134 Meet Tamia Washington Hill – She and Husband Grant Hill Open Up About MS on EXTRA, http://staging.nationalmssociety.org/online-community/personal-stories/tamia/index.aspx

noticed stamina and balance improvements, but using Betaseron provoked the activation of psoriasis, a side effect he did not like.

David does special MS Society-approved[135] exercises to help him with his gait, which he sometimes has trouble with. He has also spoken about some socially embarrassing situations caused by MS that he could not detail because no one knew he had it yet. Dropping things and falling down were just part of the ride.

These days David strongly advocates the use of disease-modifying drugs as they have worked exceptionally well in his body. He also tries to eat right and takes an active role in generating awareness for MS through public speaking and his new book, *Fall Down Laughing*.

Even with 15 years of living with MS, David continues to work, and he now owns a percentage of the Portland Beavers and is scouting for the Seattle Mariners baseball team. Between this and promoting his book, his life is still very busy. He believes in keeping things normal despite being diagnosed.

Sometimes this means using fame to educate other people, which is a big part of his life. He wants MS patients to know that with supportive diet and exercise—and the use of medication—disease symptoms do not have to progress.

Hal Ketchum: Positive Thinking and Medication

Hal Ketchum is another exceptional country music star who released more than 10 studio albums, and he regularly features on top song charts. Hal broke onto the scene with his song, "Small Town Saturday Night," and continued to create hits for several years.

Then in 1998 he was diagnosed with MS. This was a particularly disturbing diagnosis as his mother had died of MS during his life. With this new disorder to manage, he had to relearn how to do simple things, like play the guitar and walk down the road.

---

135 Squiggy Has Multiple Sclerosis, http://www.msstrength.com/squiggy-has-multiple-sclerosis/comment-page-1/

He is now 60 years old and paints, is a master carpenter, and loves to make toys for kids. Before he was diagnosed, he had trouble with his vision and speech and once had to stop playing the guitar on stage because of his illness.

Hal immediately went on MS injections three times a week. It took him a year to retrain his brain after an additional diagnosis of ARM, or acute transverse myelitis. He lost the feeling on the left side of his body, and he could not walk for a long time.

There were days when finding the energy to stand and use two canes to walk 25 feet was a good day. Despite these challenges, Hal did relearn the guitar and even performed again in his later years at the Opry. He was often called "the best voice in country music."

Painting helped him get through the worst days of his illness. These days Hal enjoys a quiet life with his family and his band. They still play music when and where possible, but Hal is sure to take his health into account first.

In many ways, after his diagnosis, longevity replaced his drive to be successful. Being ill made him realize that what matters is who you love, who you take care of, and who you go home to.[136] That is what life is all about, according to Hal Ketchum.

---

136 Tom Roland, Ketchum Takes a Healthy Approach, http://www.mult-sclerosis.org/news/Jun2003/MoreonHalKetchum.html

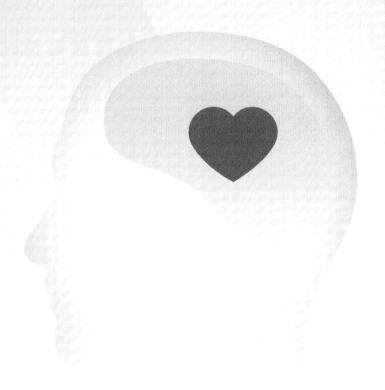

CHAPTER **15**

MS Hacking: Your Recovery Blueprint

"In life, finding a voice is speaking and living the truth. Each of you is an original. Each of you has a distinctive voice. When you find it, your story will be told. You will be heard."

JOHN GRISHAM

As someone who is recovering from multiple sclerosis and looking for unique methods of controlling, reducing, or eliminating your symptoms, you cannot do any better for yourself than a customized recovery blueprint that works best for you.

Because MS symptoms are different for everyone, you need to decide on the course of action that you are going to take to speed along your recovery. That means being open to becoming a bit of a guinea pig yourself for a while. It works!

Starting With a Personal Health Audit

To correctly formulate your own recovery blueprint, like I did, you will need to conduct an initial personal health audit. That means checking some things off your list and making sure that your health regimen is working for you.

Begin with your diagnosis. Speak with your doctor about all of your treatment options, and focus on what the repercussions of selecting those options might be. If you have side effects, what other parts of your body will suffer? Get all of the facts.

Then, audit your lifestyle. Grab a book, an Excel spreadsheet, or an app, and keep track of *how* you live. What do you eat? How does it make you feel? Record your emotions, cognitive function, and physical challenges. Notice how foods provoke certain outcomes during your three- to four-week data capture session. You can usually tell within that time.

Finally, review all of your data that you have put together for yourself. Are there any patterns? Are there foods that cause pain? Weakness? Are there activities that cause any distress? My advice would be to lay it all out and identify any correlations.

It is also a good idea to get a full blood screening from your doctor so that you can figure out if you have any food allergies or sensitivities and structure your diet accordingly. Remember that MS causes more damage in the first year[137] than in consecutive years if managed well.

Living Strategically: Setting Your Health Goals

Living strategically is how I ensure that I am looking after my health and using self-care to keep me on track with my treatments. It is easy to derail when food and exercise are large parts of your treatment regimen. You have been programmed to believe that these are not as important as they really are. But MS has changed that all for you now.

Once your personal health audit has been completed and you have at least three weeks' worth of your own habits and trials, you can get to work setting initial goals for yourself based on the severity of your symptoms.

If you need to restructure your nutritional profile, for example, this needs to become a priority—at least for the first three months

---

137 How Is MS Treated?, http://www.multiplesclerosis.com/us/treatment.php

until it feels natural. It is a huge adjustment from eating whatever you like and will require support and focus. Set your two-week sugar, wheat, and gluten detox goal and achieve it. Then set your three-month lifestyle change.

Every single day, without fail, you must be working towards a goal. That goal is to reduce or eliminate your symptoms. You should try not to cheat, as treatment with nutrition does not work if you are flooding your body with environmental toxins.

With your exercise plan, you need a solid routine. Regularity becomes your best friend when you have MS. If I skip an exercise day, I feel it. Maintaining good health is the most direct route to keeping your symptoms at bay, so make sure that you establish exercise goals and positive routines to pull you out of under or over activity.

Living strategically always takes how you feel into account. I highly recommend purchasing a biometric bracelet or health monitor[138] to count your steps, record your heart rate, and calculate how much physical activity you are getting. Review how you feel, and perfect your recovery strategy.

Implementing and Testing Practices

As you know, I have spent years testing out different diets and trying out new techniques to reduce my MS symptoms and improve my quality of life. This is what MS drives you to do. You will feel similarly compelled, which is why you stopped to purchase this book.

Because there is no cure, you should constantly seek to improve on your own recovery regimen. That means finding out which foods, exercises, or alternative therapies work best with your symptoms. It will involve an ongoing testing process.

---

138 Susan Hall, Biometric Bracelet Could Send Remote-Monitoring Data to EHRs, http://www.fiercehealthit.com/story/biometric-bracelet-could-send-remote-monitoring-data-ehrs/2012-08-09

New things will come to light all the time, and these need to be investigated. Bee Sting Therapy,[139] for example, sounds really out there at first—but many people have had success with it. You have to be fearless in your pursuit for what works.

I suggest using basic testing protocols—establish your hypothesis or what it is you are testing for, then apply it to a limited time and record the data. Then conduct a control test by staying away from that food item or exercise for the same time period.

At the end of the test, you will see how adding that element made you feel. If it improves your health a lot, it should become part of your permanent recovery strategy. For example, if you love red meat but it tends to make you feel sick, this needs to be explored.

Spend two or three weeks eating red meat often, and record your findings. Then spend three weeks not eating red meat of any kind. Notice if there are changes to your cognition, physical capabilities, and emotional state—they all count. These ongoing tests are necessary in the beginning, and you can work with a dietician to get them 100% on target.

Recording and Monitoring Your Progress

To adequately establish a pattern of routine care,[140] you need to record and monitor your progress. The enlightening thing about this is that it prevents you from consuming foods that trigger relapses, and it forces you to stay active and in shape.

My advice would be to record your progress in a journal, spreadsheet, or app of some kind, where reviewing your data will be easy. Once you have recorded all of this data, you can look at it as a whole and make deductions based on fact. Do not be afraid to detail

---

139 Background Facts: Bee Sting Therapy and MS, http://health.howstuffworks.com/medicine/tests-treatment/bee-sting-therapy-and-ms.htm

140 Rosalind Kalb, Barbara Giesser, Multiple Sclerosis: Establish a Pattern of Routine Care, http://www.dummies.com/how-to/content/multiple-sclerosis-establish-a-pattern-of-routine-.html

how you feel or what has happened to you.

After your initial audit and tests, you should continue to keep a journal that outlines your food intake, nutrient profile, and exercise regimen. It should also outline your stress management options, your supplementation regime, and any group support—if that is what you want.

That way if you suddenly spiral into an attack, you can quickly look back at what you have done differently that could have caused it. "I ate out last night, and the only viable culprit is the dish I chose; do not order it again." These insights can be as simple or as complex as you like. As always, monitoring how you feel helps your doctors too.

You can take your journals to your neurologist, your physician, and your dietician, and they will all be able to review what is happening to you and make more accurate decisions based on your details. This might sound like hard work, but the truth of the matter is that having MS is hard work, and this process gives you room to live freely again.

That is why I am a firm believer in monitoring yourself. At the end of every month at least, look back at your habits and see where you can improve. Adding improvements is a nice way to keep yourself motivated.

Always Reaching for the Cure

Currently, there is no cure for multiple sclerosis. While it is perfectly feasible to live a full and happy life with MS, it makes sense to keep an eye out for clinical trials, new drugs, and any new treatments or cures that happen to come on to the market.

You should never give up on finding a cure. As you research new treatments to test out and new foods to try, the hope should always be alive that one day your MS will go into complete remission or will be cured.

Because MS comes and goes for most patients, being vigilant about this is important. It is easy to slide back into old habits and to stop eating well and exercising regularly. But this is when attacks happen, and a bad attack can leave you in permanent disability. Your goal is to keep them at bay and to live in a permanent state of remission, as I do.

If this means subscribing to specific blogs and news outlets online, then so be it. You need to hear about these things as they happen, not years later. The American media can shut out a lot from Europe, and this could cause you to miss out on MS-free time.

That is why I make an effort every week to sit down and check if any new research, studies, tests, or breakthroughs have happened in the field—for both conventional and alternative MS treatments. When you are always on high alert for this cure, I believe you will find it first.

There are people online right now that claim to have cured their MS.[141] These individuals should be investigated but taken with a pinch of salt. Remember that MS cases vary in severity, and even if they did cure their own MS, there is no guarantee that the methods, drugs, or processes they used will work for you. Especially if they are selling something!

Taking Action When Flare-Ups Happen

When you have been diagnosed with the more common kind of MS, an attack or flare-up can happen at any time. You can go for years with the same symptoms and then just as suddenly everything will change. When flare-ups do happen, you need to take action.

Review your MS recovery strategy and journals to see what environmental influence might have triggered the response. You will know your MS has flared up when you get new symptoms that you

---

141 The Woman Who Cured Multiple Sclerosis, https://medium.com/cured-disease-naturally/the-woman-who-cured-multiple-sclerosis-11d2ebe47162

have never had before, a regular issue gets worse, or your symptoms last for longer than 24 hours.[142]

When you do experience an attack, you must treat it immediately. That means calling your doctor and searching online to see what options you have. Sometimes things like cold showers and relaxation can do a lot to help worsening symptoms.

Either way, if you are conscientious in keeping a record of your habits, you might be able to identify the things that are triggering you. Then you can cut them out. By noticing, for example, that on the last three separate occasions, your symptoms seemed to get worse when you ate a tomato-based dish, this may mean that tomatoes could trigger your MS.

No one is going to do this research and monitoring for you; it has to be something that you take on personally so that you can reduce the frequency of your attacks. If you cannot figure out why an attack has happened, or it continues to linger and progress, see you doctor.

If at any point your symptoms get seriously bad, you will need to go on medication. This can help reduce the frequency of your attacks, but it will result in horrible side effects. That is why you have to be vigilant with yourself and stick to your treatment routine.

Building a Supportive Environment

As someone with MS, getting by on a day-to-day basis is going to be hard. Some days will be better than others, but the reality is that you have to live with a serious illness until a cure is found. That means you will need a highly supportive environment where you can feel safe and are able to practice your recovery routine daily.

Family and friends will need to understand that your new lifestyle changes are critical to your physical, emotional, and mental wellbeing. They will not understand at first, and many may try to talk

---

142 Gina Shaw, Treat and Prevent a Multiple Sclerosis Flare-Up, http://www.webmd.com/multiple-sclerosis/features/flare-ups

you into drinking, eating, and behaving as you once did. However, this is not going to benefit you and may even cause an MS relapse.

It is important that your family habits change with yours because that is what real support looks like. Ideally, you want to eat the same things to guarantee your ongoing recovery. That means that your family should consider making the lifestyle changes too; it can only benefit them. That way you will not feel alone in your struggle.

Alternatively, you can try to find a local MS support group.[143] While I have not had any success with groups myself and find that many of them are funded by the pharmaceutical companies, which is not ideal, you might decide to start a group of your own with other MS patients in your area.

It can be constructive to share experiences with other MS patients as well as treatment results and insight. I have friends who have MS, and they are very dear to me. Even though I know that their MS is different from mine, listening to friends has led me to discover many valuable things about the disease I did not know before. All of it has led to my recovery.

Speed Dial: Your Help Infrastructure

When bad symptoms strike and you need help, you need multiple methods of calling for it. I have found that making it easy to contact essential people and places is a critical part of my treatment plan. MS patients are clumsy; we fall, and we drop things. Injuries are not uncommon, and there may be a time when you need help on speed dial.

- Make sure that your spouse is on speed dial or your next of kin. You should only have to press two things to contact them in case of emergency.

---

143 Kimberly Holland, Multiple Sclerosis Support Groups, http://www.healthline.com/health-slideshow/multiple-sclerosis-support-groups

- Add your local emergency room numbers to your speed dial list, or if your MS has become particularly bad, have an emergency alarm placed in your home.
- Your neurologist's number should also be on this list along with two other backup physicians that you can call if an emergency strikes and your doctor is not available.
- Ambulance and health insurance numbers can also be placed here, or you can use an app to store all of your personal medical information in case of emergency.

Start by compiling a list of important people and places related to your MS, and draft methods of contacting them—whether it is via email, phone call, or instant message. Your support group members can also be on this list for the times you are feeling low and need some encouragement and support.

Sit down with your family and discuss with your kids what you should do if something happens. Explain where to find the emergency numbers and how to get help there if you are unable to make the call yourself. This prepares you for any eventuality.

Consistent Evaluation and Doctors' Visits

Once you are diagnosed and have started your treatment regimen, your doctor will want to monitor your progress regularly. That means making yourself available for consistent evaluation and any number of doctors' visits for screenings and checks.

Try to find a neurologist that is willing to work with you on your natural treatment regimen and that has an open mind about alternative therapies. Prepare for each appointment by creating a list of questions that you may have about your disease or symptoms.

Make sure to outline everything that you want to talk about—even the sensitive subjects. All MS patients need a caring healthcare practitioner that will facilitate the recovery process. This means introducing your physician to your neurologist and any other doctors that have had an opinion on your symptoms or diagnosis.

Keeping in regular contact with your doctors is important[144] because they will help provide you with treatment options in case of worsening symptoms, and they will send you to have additional MRIs to check on your lesion progression.

When you are consistently evaluated, you will gain additional diagnostic evidence to either support or refuse your own personal MS recovery treatment. There are people in the world that have pitched up to MRIs with reduced lesions and fewer signs of MS progression.

If you do not show up and engage with your doctor regularly, you will miss out on valuable insight. That said, it is essential that you find an open minded doctor. Some neurologists are set in their ways and will not treat you if you do not take the medication that they prescribe.

Make the most of each visit by being prepared and learning something new each time you go. Your doctor is not only a treatment professional but an excellent knowledge resource and someone with lots of experience with other MS cases.

Your Personal MS Recovery Story

Sticking with your customized recovery strategy and treatment plan will work wonders for your independence, your self-esteem, and the way in which you view this disease. It does not define who you are, but it does give you more challenges than most people.

This means that you have the opportunity to care for yourself in ways most people do not think about until they are my age! Your body really is a temple, and you should treat it like sacred ground to keep your MS symptoms at bay.

---

144 Make the Most of Your Doctor Visits, http://www.nationalmssociety.org/Treating-MS/Comprehensive-Care/Make-the-Most-of-Your-Doctor-Visits

If you can embrace these lifestyle changes and truly formulate a recovery strategy for yourself, I believe that it will work for you the same way it worked for me. I am older now—and wiser—and have realized that when life leaves you without a cure, it does not leave you without options. There are always actions that you can take to help yourself.

This is how you will write your own personal MS recovery story. I urge you that when the time comes to share this story with the world, you let others know about this route, as I have. I believe that one by one, MS patients can inform and educate themselves and lead healthy, happy lives with their loved ones.

The only thing standing in your way is gone; now you have the knowledge and the evidence needed to take action. The rest is a matter of trusting yourself, doing the work, and putting in the consistent effort. MS does not go away, so learning to control it will give you the power you need to stay positive until a cure arrives.

In the meantime, keep your family close, and believe in yourself. You did not choose to have MS in your life, but you can choose to make the most of the life you have been privileged enough to be given. Appreciate what you have, be grateful for the action you can take, and trust that soon things will be better.

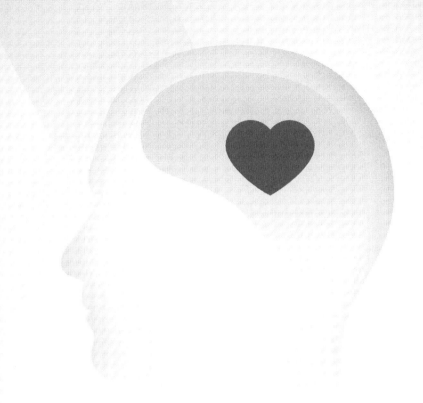

Conclusion

The beginning of your personal MS recovery story begins now. Soon you will be an inspiration to others and will have the ability to spread the word about adequate nutrition, exercise, alternative treatments, and the importance of self-care.

Do not dwell on the fact that there is no cure as of yet. Millions of dollars are being channeled into research, and there are thousands of people all over the globe working hard to find one. That is their job—yours is to save your own life.

I may not know your circumstances—or how MS has impacted your life—but I know that you have the power to change the way that you live so that MS does not overwhelm you. And on those days when you cannot find any rest and everything seems haywire, I want you to focus on the positive and keep treating yourself.

Recovery does not happen overnight, but it is a routine that needs to survive for quite some time before it works efficiently. I have seen MS from the perspective of a doctor and a patient and have come to this conclusion:

Let the healthcare professionals find the answer while you focus on your own recovery. Build a supportive healthcare team that will fuel instead of stunt your investigations. Be open to trying new things, but do not be hesitant to stop them if they hurt you. Your body is an amazing test subject, and it will reward you for listening.

Multiple sclerosis is not the end of your life but the beginning of a fuller life, where your emotional, physical, and mental needs have got to come first. If you can master yourself, you will master this disease!

Keep the faith,

Cynthia Guy, MD

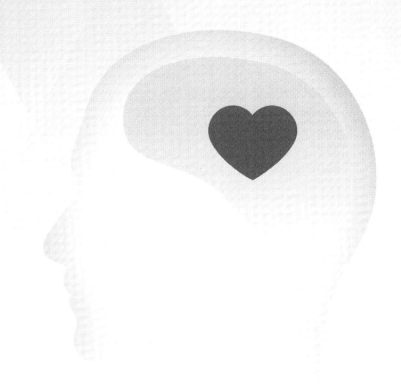

FREE SPECIAL BONUS

Thank you so much for purchasing and reading this book. As a special bonus for readers, I am offering a free Get Healthy Plan covering the stages of health outlined in this book, a gluten-free shopping list, recipes and more!

Download your guide instantly at http://www.nutrilifewellness. com/love-yourself-healthy-bonus

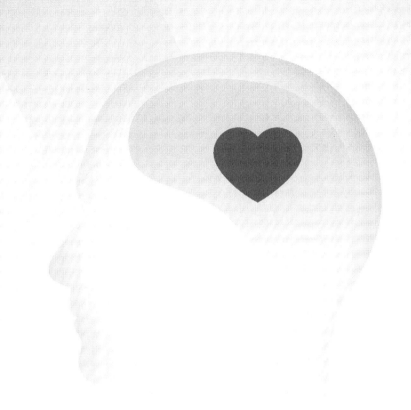

References

Chapter 1

MS Quotes, http://www.brainyquote.com/quotes/keywords/ms.html

Multiple Sclerosis Health Center Treatment And Care, http://www.webmd.com/multiple-sclerosis/guide/multiple-sclerosis-treatment-care

Multiple Sclerosis, http://www.nytimes.com/health/guides/disease/multiple-sclerosis/overview.html

Treating MS, http://www.nationalmssociety.org/Treating-MS

Signs And Symptoms, http://www.mssociety.org.uk/what-is-ms/signs-and-symptoms

Gardner, Amanda, Could you have MS? 16 Multiple Sclerosis Symptoms, http://www.foxnews.com/health/2013/07/16/could-have-ms-16-multiple-sclerosis-symptoms/

Recognize Multiple Sclerosis Symptoms, http://www.webmd.com/multiple-sclerosis/guide/multiple-sclerosis-diagnosis

Pietrangelo, Ann, Multiple Sclerosis From Top To Bottom Getting The Complete Picture, http://www.healthline.com/health/multiple-sclerosis/effects-on-the-body

What Are The Symptoms And Effects Of Multiple Sclerosis? http://www.imaginis.com/multiple-sclerosis-symptoms-diagnosis/what-are-the-symptoms-and-effects-of-multiple-sclerosis

Sullivan, Amy, Psy.D, The Psychological Impact Of MS, http://my.clevelandclinic.org/multimedia/transcripts/psychological-impact-of-multiple-sclerosis.aspx

Medscape, http://www.medscape.org/viewarticle/734647

Chwastiak, Lydia, A, Ehde, Dawn, M, Psychiatric Issues In Multiple Sclerosis, http://www.ncbi.nlm.nih.gov/pmc/articles/PMC2706287/

Rickards, Hugh, Abnormal Mental States In Multiple Sclerosis, http://www.mstrust.org.uk/professionals/information/wayahead/articles/07012003_02.jsp

Emotional Changes, http://www.nationalmssociety.org/Symptoms-Diagnosis/MS-Symptoms/Emotional-Changes

Emotions, http://www.mssociety.org.uk/what-is-ms/signs-and-symptoms/mental-health/emotions

Chapter 2

Quotes About Multiple Sclerosis, http://www.goodreads.com/quotes/tag/multiple-sclerosis

Multiple Sclerosis Resources In The World 2008, http://www.who.int/mental_health/neurology/Atlas_MS_WEB.pdf

Treating Multiple Sclerosis, http://www.nhs.uk/Conditions/Multiple-sclerosis/Pages/Treatment.aspx

Caring For Someone With Multiple Sclerosis, http://www.nhs.uk/CarersDirect/guide/kinds/Pages/caring-for-someone-with-multiple-sclerosis.aspx

Call Therapy For Multiple Sclerosis Patients: Closer Than Ever? http://www.sciencedaily.com/news/health_medicine/multiple_sclerosis/

New Blood Cells Fight Brain Inflammation, http://www.sciencedaily.com/releases/2014/02/140216151715.htm

Education Attenuates Impact Of TBI On Cognition, http://www.sciencedaily.com/releases/2014/02/140228121357.htm

Medical Marijuana May Ease Some MS; Little Evidence For Other Complementary Or Alternative Therapies, http://www.sciencedaily.com/releases/2014/03/140324181258.htm

Stem Cells From Muscle Can Repair Nerve Damage After Injury, http://www.sciencedaily.com/releases/2014/03/140318190035.htm

Bacterial Toxin Potential Trigger For Multiple Sclerosis, http://www.sciencedaily.com/releases/2014/01/140128153940.htm

Monajem, Roya, Meeting Of Eastern-Western Medicine: A Possible Alternative Treatment For Multiple Sclerosis, http://www.payvand.com/news/09/apr/1103.html

Western Medicine Multiple Sclerosis (MS) Information, http://www.yinyanghouse.com/treatments/multiple_sclerosis_healthinfo

Hollingsworth, Catherine, Treating Multiple Sclerosis With Chinese Medicine, http://www.acupuncturetoday.com/mpacms/at/article.php?id=32721

MS Diagnosis, http://www.ms-uk.org/MSdiagnosis

Rolak, Loren, A, The History Of MS, http://www.nationalmssociety.org/NationalMSSociety/media/MSNationalFiles/Brochures/Brochure-History-of-Multiple-Sclerosis.pdf

Murray, Jock, T, Multiple Sclerosis: The History Of A Disease, http://www.ncbi.nlm.nih.gov/pmc/articles/PMC1142241/

Roth, Erica, The History Of Multiple Sclerosis: How Far Have We come? http://www.healthline.com/health-slideshow/history-multiple-sclerosis-how-far-have-we-come#promoSlide

What Causes MS? http://www.nationalmssociety.org/What-is-MS/What-Causes-MS

What Causes Multiple Sclerosis, http://www.webmd.com/multiple-sclerosis/guide/multiple-sclerosis-causes

Diagnosing Tools, http://www.nationalmssociety.org/Symptoms-Diagnosis/Diagnosing-Tools

The Tests For MS, http://www.mssociety.org.uk/what-is-ms/information-about-ms/diagnosis/tests-for-ms

Multiple Sclerosis Diagnosis And Tests, http://www.webmd.com/multiple-sclerosis/guide/multiple-sclerosis-diagnosis-tests

Steenhuysen, Julie, High Salt Diets May Be Behind Rising Autoimmune Disease Rates, Studies Find, http://www.huffingtonpost.com/2013/03/06/salt-autoimmune-disease-sodium-multiple-sclerosis-diabetes_n_2821200.html

Autoimmune Statistics, http://www.aarda.org/autoimmune-information/autoimmune-statistics/

Okada, H, Kuhn, C, Feillet, H, Bach, J, F, The 'Hygiene Hypothesis' For Autoimmune And Allergic Diseases: An Update, http://www.ncbi.nlm.nih.gov/pmc/articles/PMC2841828/

Guthrie, Catherine. Autoimmune Disorders: When Your Body Turns On You, http://experiencelife.com/article/autoimmune-disorders-when-your-body-turns-on-you/

What Is Multiple Sclerosis, http://www.webmd.com/multiple-sclerosis/guide/what-is-multiple-sclerosis

Definition Of Multiple Sclerosis, http://www.nationalmssociety.org/What-is-MS/Definition-of-MS

Chapter 3

MS Quotes, http://www.brainyquote.com/quotes/keywords/ms.html

Healthline Editorial Team, Early Signs Of Multiple Sclerosis, http://www.healthline.com/health-slideshow/multiple-sclerosis

Recognize Multiple Sclerosis Symptoms, http://www.webmd.com/multiple-sclerosis/guide/multiple-sclerosis-diagnosis

Recognizing Multiple Sclerosis Symptoms, http://www.webmd.com/multiple-sclerosis/guide/multiple-sclerosis-symptoms-types

Could You Have MS? 16 Multiple Sclerosis Symptoms, http://www.health.com/health/gallery/0,,20639076_2,00.html

Multiple Sclerosis, http://www.nytimes.com/health/guides/disease/multiple-sclerosis/symptoms.html

Multiple Sclerosis And Fatigue, http://www.webmd.com/multiple-sclerosis/guide/ms-related-fatigue

Potts, Alison, It's Like Being Switched Off, http://www.bbc.com/news/health-18207490

Numbness Or Tingling, http://www.nationalmssociety.org/Symptoms-Diagnosis/MS-Symptoms/Numbness

Numbness, http://www.mymsaa.org/about-ms/symptoms/numbness/

Numbness Or Tingling, http://multiplesclerosis.net/symptoms/numbness-tingling/

Causes Of Balance And Walking Problems, http://www.mssociety.org.uk/what-is-ms/signs-and-symptoms/balance-and-dizziness/causes

Glossary Of MS Terms, http://www.mslifelines.com/pages/what-is-ms/glossary#spasticity

Coping With Multiple Sclerosis, http://www.msfocus.org/article-details.aspx?articleID=511

Sarkan, N, B, Involuntary Movements In Multiple Sclerosis, http://www.ncbi.nlm.nih.gov/pmc/articles/PMC1991657/

Abnormal Involuntary Movements, http://www.patient.co.uk/doctor/Abnormal-Involuntary-Movements.htm

Schneyder, N, Harris, M, K, Minagar, A, Movement Disorders In Patients With Multiple Sclerosis, http://www.ncbi.nlm.nih.gov/pubmed/21496590

Controlling the Muscle Spasms Of Multiple Sclerosis, http://www.webmd.com/multiple-sclerosis/guide/controlling-muscle-spasms

Shin, Rovert, MD, Focusing On Visual Disturbance Of MS, http://www.msfocus.org/article-details.aspx?articleID=808

Multiple Sclerosis And Vision Problems, http://www.webmd.com/multiple-sclerosis/guide/multiple-sclerosis-vision-problems

Speech Problems, http://www.nationalmssociety.org/Symptoms-Diagnosis/MS-Symptoms/Speech-Disorders

Pain, http://www.nationalmssociety.org/Symptoms-Diagnosis/MS-Symptoms/Pain

Shaw, Gina, Treating Multiple Sclerosis Pain, http://www.webmd.com/multiple-sclerosis/guide/treating-multiple-sclerosis-pain

Could You Have MS? 16 Multiple Sclerosis Symptoms, http://www.health.com/health/gallery/0,,20639076_8,00.html

Bladder Problems, http://www.nationalmssociety.org/Symptoms-Diagnosis/MS-Symptoms/Bladder-Dysfunction

Multiple Sclerosis And Bowel Problems, http://www.webmd.com/multiple-sclerosis/guide/bowel-problem-linked

Bowel Problems, http://www.nationalmssociety.org/Symptoms-Diagnosis/MS-Symptoms/Bowel-Problems

Sexual Dysfunction, http://www.nationalmssociety.org/Symptoms-Diagnosis/MS-Symptoms/Sexual-Dysfunction

Emrich, Lisa, Sexual Dysfunction And Multiple Sclerosis, http://www.healthcentral.com/multiple-sclerosis/c/19065/71212/sexual/

Cognitive Changes, http://www.nationalmssociety.org/Symptoms-Diagnosis/MS-Symptoms/Cognitive-Changes

Cognitive And Emotional Changes, http://www.msif.org/about-ms/symptoms/congitive-and-mood-changes.aspx

Chapter 4

MS Quotations, http://msquotations.com/

Renter, Elizabeth, 'Mainstream' Doctors And Nurses Often Use Alternative Medicine For Themselves, http://naturalsociety.com/doctors-and-nurses-often-prefer-alternative-medicine/

Western Medicine Is 'Reductionist', http://www.insightcenter.net/articles/western-medicine-is-reductionist/

Holism vs. Reductionism: Comparing The Fundamentals Of Conventional And Alternative Medicinal Modalities, http://exploreim.ucla.edu/education/holism-vs-reductionism-comparing-the-fundamentals-of-conventional-and-alternative-medicinal-modalities/

Beresford, Mark, J, Medical Reductionism: Lessons From The Philosophers, http://qjmed.oxfordjournals.org/content/103/9/721.long

Common Side Effects OF MS Medication, http://www.msactivesource.com/side_effects.xml

Parikh, Rahul, Why Does Your Doctor Hate Alternative Medicine? http://www.salon.com/2011/05/02/alternative_medicine_and_doctors_oz/

Anderson, Sylvia, Why Do These People Hate Alternative Medicine/ http://www.insidershealth.com/article/why_do_these_people_hate_alternative_medicine/5005

Schwager, Sarah, War Against Natural Medicine, http://www.abc.net.au/unleashed/3840682.html

Doctor's Don't Follow Their Own Advice On Medical Treatment, http://gizmodo.com/5976978/doctors-dont-want-treatment-even-when-theyre-dying

Koren, Marina, America Is Running Out Of Doctors, http://www.nationaljournal.com/health-care/america-is-running-out-of-doctors-20131104

Parker-Pope, Tara, When A Doctor Plays Down Your Symptoms, http://well.blogs.nytimes.com/2010/04/12/when-a-doctor-downplays-your-symptoms/?_php=true&_type=blogs&_r=0

Grady, Denise, In Reporting Symptoms, Don't Patients Know Best? http://www.nytimes.com/2010/04/13/health/13seco.html?ref=health

Getting A Diagnosis, http://www.msfocus.org/being-diagnosed.aspx

Coping With Multiple Sclerosis, http://www.msfocus.org/article-details.aspx?articleID=344

Stachowiak, Julie, Reader Response: Describe Your 'MS Journey', Diagnosis Of Multiple Sclerosis,http://ms.about.com/u/ua/readermsstoriesandtips/Diagnosis-Of-Multiple-Sclerosis-Stories-About-Being-Diagnosed-With-Multiple-Sclerosis.htm

Chapter 5

MS Quotations, http://msquotations.com/

Roth, Erica, 5 Promising New Treatments For MS, http://www.healthline.com/health-slideshow/5-promising-new-treatments-ms#7

Randomized Trial Of Oral Teriflunomide For Relapsing Multiple Sclerosis, http://www.nejm.org/doi/full/10.1056/NEJMoa1014656

Multiple Sclerosis And 'Miracle Cures': Sometimes It's The Hope that'll Kill You, http://www.theguardian.com/science/brain-flapping/2014/apr/17/multiple-sclerosis-miracle-cures-ms

Zamboni, Paolo, The Big Idea: Iron-Dependent Inflammation In Venous Disease And Proposed Parallels In Multiple Sclerosis, http://jrs.sagepub.com/content/99/11/589.long

Watson, Stephanie, CCSVI And Multiple Sclerosis, http://www.webmd.com/multiple-sclerosis/features/ccsvi-and-multiple-sclerosis

What Is CCSVI? http://www.ccsvi.org/index.php/the-basics/what-is-ccsvi

Randomized Controlled Trial Of Yoga And Exercise In Multiple Sclerosis, http://www.uvm.edu/~rsingle/JournalClub/papers/Oken%2BNeurology-2004_MS%2Byoga.pdf

Welcome To The Yoga Jungle, http://www.nationalmssociety.org/Living-Well-With-MS/Health-Wellness/Exercise/Yoga

Are There Any Natural Remedies For Multiple Sclerosis? http://www.drweil.com/drw/u/QAA35890/Natural-Remedies-For-Multiple-Sclerosis.html

A Controversial 'Cure' For MS, http://www.nytimes.com/2012/10/28/magazine/a-controversial-cure-for-multiple-sclerosis.html?pagewanted=2

Groundbreaking Multiple Sclerosis Stem Cell Trial Approved, http://www.medicalnewstoday.com/articles/264892.php

Stem Cell Therapy, http://www.mssociety.org.uk/ms-research/new-and-potential-treatments/stem-cell-therapy

Side Effects of MS Treatments, http://www.webmd.com/multiple-sclerosis/features/ms-side-effects?page=2

Complementary & Alternative Medicine, http://www.nationalmssociety.org/Treating-MS/Complementary-Alternative-Medicines

Complementary And Alternative Medicine, http://www.mstrust.org.uk/atoz/cam.jsp

Brind'Amour, Katie, Going Herbal: Vitamins And Supplements For Multiple Sclerosis, http://www.healthline.com/health/multiple-sclerosis/going-herbal-vitamins-and-supplements-for-multiple-sclerosis#3

MS Drug Continues To Cause Disastrous Side Effects, http://articles.mercola.com/sites/articles/archive/2010/02/25/ms-drug-continues-to-cause-disastrous-side-effects.aspx

Diet, http://www.ms-uk.org/dietresearch

Eck, Deborah, The Supplement Maze, http://www.msfocus.org/article-details.aspx?articleID=459

Summary Of Evidence-Based Guidelines: Complementary And Alternative Medicine In Multiple Sclerosis, http://www.msif.org/global-ms-research/latest-ms-research-news/summary-of-evidence-based-guidelines-complementary-and-alternative-medicine-in-multiple-sclerosis.aspx

Latest MS Research News, http://www.msif.org/global-ms-research/latest-ms-research-news/

Emerging Areas Of Research, http://www.mssociety.org.uk/ms-research/emerging-areas

Chapter 6

You Can Do It Quotes, http://www.brainyquote.com/quotes/keywords/you_can_do_it.html

Dirt Poor: Have Fruits And Vegetables Become Less Nutritious? http://www.scientificamerican.com/article/soil-depletion-and-nutrition-loss/

Schwarz, Stefan, Leweling, Hans, Multiple Sclerosis And Nutrition, http://www.pinnaclife.com/sites/default/files/research/MS_and_Nutrition.pdf

The MS Diet, http://www.msdietforwomen.com/ms-diet

Diet And Multiple Sclerosis (MS) Information, http://www.second-opinions.co.uk/foods-and-ms.html#.U5xkLfmSySo

Ashtari, Fereshteh, Jamshidi, Fatemeh, Shoormasti, Raheleh, Shokouhi, Pourpak, Zahra, and Akbari, Mojtaba, Cow's Milk Allergy In Multiple Sclerosis Patients, http://www.ncbi.nlm.nih.gov/pmc/articles/PMC3743324/

The Food Guide Pyramid, http://www.cnpp.usda.gov/publications/mypyramid/originalfoodguidepyramids/fgp/fgppamphlet.pdf

Selig, Meg, Why Diets Don't Work … And What Does, http://www.psychologytoday.com/blog/changepower/201010/why-diets-dont-workand-what-does

5 Reasons Most Diets Fail Within 7 Days, http://www.huffingtonpost.com/2013/09/24/why-diets-dont-work_n_3975610.html

Jordan, Jo, How To Use Food Combining Techniques For Better Digestion, http://www.puristat.com/bloating/Food-Combining.aspx

Adamson, Eve, Lifestyle V. Diet: Pick A Side, http://strongertogether.coop/food-lifestyle/lifestyle-v-diet/

Young, Lisa, Lifestyle Intervention Beats Diet For Weight Loss: 6 Simple Changes To Make Today, http://www.huffingtonpost.com/dr-lisa-young/lifestyle-weight-loss_b_3831981.html

Sarah, Milk And MS, http://www.macrobiotic.org/msmilk.html

McCoy, Krisha, The Macrobiotic Diet, http://www.everydayhealth.com/diet-nutrition/macrobiotic-diet.aspx

Macrobiotic Diet, http://www.webmd.com/diet/macrobiotic-diet

Raw Foods Diet, http://www.webmd.com/diet/raw-foods-diet

The Nature Of Change, http://mindsetonline.com/changeyourmindset/natureofchange/

Hyman, Mark, Dr, Sweet Poison: How Sugar, Not Cocaine, Is One Of The Most Addictive And Dangerous Substances, http://www.nydailynews.com/life-style/health/white-poison-danger-sugar-beat-article-1.1605232

Chapter 7

15 Health And Nutrition Inspirational Quotes, http://www.obesityhelp.com/articles/15-health-and-nutrition-inspirational-quotes

Michaelis, Kristin, Healthy Meats: What To Buy, http://www.foodrenegade.com/healthy-meats-what-to-buy/

The Best Protein Choices And Worst For Your Health And The Environment, http://www.eatingwell.com/food_news_origins/green_sustainable/best_meat_worst_meat_the_best_protein_choices

Sarah, The Home Economist, 170 Scientific Studies Confirm The Dangers Of Soy, http://www.thehealthyhomeeconomist.com/170-scientific-reasons-to-lose-the-soy-in-your-diet/

Philpott, Tom, Monsanto GM Soy Is Scarier Than You Think, http://www.motherjones.com/tom-philpott/2014/04/superweeds-arent-only-trouble-gmo-soy

Blood Sugar Balance And Multiple Sclerosis, https://www.theholisticdirectory.co.uk/articles/story/blood-sugar-balance-and-ms

The Truth About Carbs, http://www.nhs.uk/Livewell/loseweight/Pages/the-truth-about-carbs.aspx

Sugar Again…The More We Learn About Multiple Sclerosis, http://www.sparkpeople.com/mypage_public_journal_individual.asp?blog_id=5332066

Richeh, Wael, Gutierrez, Amparo, Lovera, Jesus, The Association Between Serum Glucose And Disability Progression In Multiple Sclerosis (PO4.130), http://www.neurology.org/cgi/content/meeting_abstract/80/1_MeetingAbstracts/P04.130

Kent, George, Food Quality: An Issue As Important As Safety, http://www.foodsafetynews.com/2012/07/food-safety-not-just-an-issue-of-immediate-threats/#.U507xvmSySo

What Not To Eat, http://www.overcomingmultiplesclerosis.org/Recovery-Program/Diet/What-Not-to-Eat/

Doctor Reverses Multiple Sclerosis In 9 Months By Eating These Foods, http://articles.mercola.com/sites/articles/archive/2011/12/23/overcoming-multiple-sclerosis-through-diet.aspx

Benito, León, J, Pisa, D, Alonso, R, Calleja, P, Díaz-Sánchez, M, Carrasco, L, Association Between Multiple Sclerosis And Candida Species: Evidence From A Case-Control Study, http://www.ncbi.nlm.nih.gov/pubmed/20556470

Dean, Carolyn, MD, ND, Yeast Gone Wild, http://www.needs.com/product/NDNL-0704-01/a_Candida

Types Of Fats, http://www.overcomingmultiplesclerosis.org/Recovery-Program/Role-of-Fats-in-MS/Types-of-Fats/

The Truth About Fats: Bad And Good, http://www.health.harvard.edu/fhg/updates/Truth-about-fats.shtml

Wong, Cathy, Candida Diet – Foods To Avoid, http://altmedicine.about.com/od/popularhealthdiets/a/candida_foods1.htm

What Causes Multiple Sclerosis? http://www.holistichelp.net/blog/what-causes-multiple-sclerosis/

Mehta, LR, Dworkin, RH, Schwid, SR, Polyunsaturated Fatty Acids And Their Potential Therapeutic Role In Multiple Sclerosis, http://www.ncbi.nlm.nih.gov/pubmed/19194388

Dehydration, http://www.ndhealthfacts.org/wiki/Dehydration

Multiple Sclerosis Lifestyle Changes, http://www.nytimes.com/health/guides/disease/multiple-sclerosis/lifestyle-changes.html

Chapter 8

Wheat Belly Quotes, https://www.goodreads.com/work/quotes/16440712-wheat-belly-lose-the-wheat-lose-the-weight-and-find-your-path-back-to

Oricessed Gluten-Free Foods Can Be Hazardous To Your Health, Not Helpful, Experts Say, http://www.post-gazette.com/frontpage/2013/11/04/DIET-S-DOWNSIDE/stories/201311040018

Reasons To Adopt A Gluten-Free Diet, http://imtwellnesscenter.com/reasons-to-adopt-a-gluten-free-diet.php

Hyman, Mark, MD, Gluten: What You Don't Know Might Kill You, http://drhyman.com/blog/2011/03/17/gluten-what-you-dont-know-might-kill-you/#close

Rettner, Rachael, Most People Shouldn't Eat Gluten-Free, http://www.scientificamerican.com/article/most-people-shouldnt-eat-gluten-free/

Davis, William, Dr, FAQ's, http://www.wheatbellyblog.com/faqs/

Hamblin, James, This Is Your Brain On Gluten, http://www.theatlantic.com/health/archive/2013/12/this-is-your-brain-on-gluten/282550/

Kerr, Michael, Gluten Allergies Food List: What To Avoid & What To Eat, http://www.healthline.com/health/allergies/gluten-food-list#2

Strawbridge, Holly, Going Gluten-Free Just Because? Here's What You Need To Know, http://www.health.harvard.edu/blog/going-gluten-free-just-because-heres-what-you-need-to-know-201302205916

Welsh, Jennifer, Researchers Who Provided Key Evidence For Gluten Sensitivity Have Now Thoroughly Shown That It Doesn't Exist, http://www.businessinsider.com/gluten-sensitivity-and-study-replication-2014-5

Ozello, Donald, A, MS And Gluten-Free Diet, http://www.livestrong.com/article/239686-ms-gluten-free-diet/

Bowling, Allen, Diet & MS: An Interview With Dr Allen Bowling, http://www.msconnection.org/Blog/June-2013/Diet-MS-An-interview-with-Dr-Allen-Bowling

What Foods Have Gluten, http://www.diabetes.org/food-and-fitness/food/planning-meals/gluten-free-diets/what-foods-have-gluten.html

Gunnars, Chris, 6 Reasons Why Gluten May Be Bad For You, http://authoritynutrition.com/6-shocking-reasons-why-gluten-is-bad/

Fasano, A, Berti, I, Gerarduzzi, T, Not, T, Colletti, RB, Drago, S, Elitsur, Y, Green, PH, Guandalini, S, Hill, ID, Pietzak, M, Ventura, A, Thorpe, M, Kryszak, D, Fornaroli, F, Wasserman, SS, Murray, JA, Horvath, K,

Prevalence Of Celiac Disease In At-Risk and Not-At-Risk Groups In The United States: A Large Multicenter Study, http://www.ncbi.nlm.nih.gov/pubmed/12578508/

Tapia, Alberto Rubio, Kyle, Robert, A, Kaplan, Edward, L, Johnson, Dwight, R, Page, William, Erdtmann, Frederick, Brantner, Tricia, L, Kim, W. Ray, Phelps, Tara K, Lahr, Brian D, Zinsmeister, Alan R, Melton III, L. Joseph, Murray, Joseph A, Increased Prevalence And Mortality In Undiagnosed Celiac Disease, http://www.gastrojournal.org/article/S0016-5085(09)00523-X/abstract

Chapter 9

Sugar, BrainyQuote, http://www.brainyquote.com/quotes/keywords/sugar.html#MbHiFOxmU8hQC2VM.99

Kornbluth, Jesse, Drop That Whole Wheat Bread! No More Cereal! Grain Brain, A#1 Bestseller, Says: 'Abandon Gluten!

http://www.huffingtonpost.com/jesse-kornbluth/drop-that-whole-wheat-bre_b_4631108.html

Hoover, Rebecca, Right Diet May Be The Best Way To Beat Multiple Sclerosis And Sizzle Too, http://intelligentguidetoms.wordpress.com/

Ritterman, Jeff, MD, Sugar Kills! How Do We Decrease Consumption? http://www.huffingtonpost.com/jeffrey-ritterman/sugar-kills-how-do-we-dec_b_4977021.html

Shaw, Kerry, Why Wheat Is Ruining Your Life: The Author Of Wheat Belly Explains, http://www.mindbodygreen.com/0-9484/why-wheat-is-ruining-your-life-the-author-of-wheat-belly-explains.html

Hook, BS, Multiple Sclerosis And Wheat (Gluten)…A Connection, http://drbradshook.com/2011/07/multiple-sclerosis-and-wheat-gluten-a-connection/

Doctor Reverses Multiple Sclerosis In 9 Months By Eating These Foods, http://articles.mercola.com/sites/articles/archive/2011/12/23/overcoming-multiple-sclerosis-through-diet.aspx

Richeh, Wael, Gutierrez, Amparo, Lovera, Jesus, The Association Between Serum Glucose Level And Disability Progression In Multiple Sclerosis

(P04.130), http://www.neurology.org/cgi/content/meeting_abstract/80/1_MeetingAbstracts/P04.130

Salt Link To Multiple Sclerosis Unproven, http://www.nhs.uk/news/2013/03March/Pages/Salt-link-to-multiple-sclerosis-unproven.aspx

Harmon, Katherine, Salt Linked To Autoimmune Diseases, http://www.nature.com/news/salt-linked-to-autoimmune-diseases-1.12555

Gallagher, James, Salt Linked To Immune Rebellion In Study, http://www.bbc.com/news/health-21685022

Americans Consume Too Much Sodium (Salt), http://www.cdc.gov/features/dssodium/

Salt Stats, http://www.cdc.gov/salt/pdfs/salt_stats_media.pdf

Anderson, Jane, Celiac Disease And Multiple Sclerosis, http://celiacdisease.about.com/od/symptomsofceliacdisease/a/Celiac-Disease-And-Multiple-Sclerosis.htm

Batur-Caglayan, HZ, Irkec, C, Yildirim-Capraz, I, Atalay-Akyurek, N, Dumlu, S, A Case Of Multiple Sclerosis And Celiac Disease, http://www.ncbi.nlm.nih.gov/pmc/articles/PMC3556850/

Study: Celiac Disease Prevalence 5 – 10 Times Higher In MS Patients, http://www.celiaccentral.org/research-news/Celiac-Disease-Research/134/month--201103/search--MS/vobid--5192/

Chapter 10

Quotes About Self Care, http://www.goodreads.com/quotes/tag/self-care

Side Effects of Medicine, http://www.mhra.gov.uk/Safetyinformation/Generalsafetyinformationandadvice/Adviceandinformationforconsumers/Sideeffectsofmedicines/

MS In Family Members, http://www.overcomingmultiplesclerosis.org/Recovery-Program/MS-in-Family-Members/

Taking Care Of You: Self-Care For Family Caregivers, https://www.caregiver.org/taking-care-you-self-care-family-caregivers

Talking To Your Family About Multiple Sclerosis, http://www.webmd.com/multiple-sclerosis/guide/ms-family

Multiple Sclerosis Family And Friend Support, http://www.mslifelines.com/pages/wellness-and-ms/family_and_friends

Rankin, Lisa, Collaboration Trumps Competition In Health Care, http://www.psychologytoday.com/blog/owning-pink/201201/collaboration-trumps-competition-in-health-care

Multiple Sclerosis (MS) – When To Call A Doctor, http://www.webmd.com/multiple-sclerosis/tc/multiple-sclerosis-ms-when-to-call-a-doctor

Woodward, Matthew, The Ninja's Guide To Google Alerts, http://www.searchenginejournal.com/the-ninjas-guide-to-google-alerts/48068/

Marcus, Mary, Brophy, Read The Labels, Because 'All Drugs Have Side Effects', http://usatoday30.usatoday.com/LIFE/usaedition/2011-08-04-Overthecounter-drug-dangers--_ST_U.htm

Side Effects Of Medicines, http://www.mhra.gov.uk/Safetyinformation/Generalsafetyinformationandadvice/Adviceandinformationforconsumers/Sideeffectsofmedicines/

Copaxone – What Dose Is Right For you? https://www.copaxone.com/about-copaxone/dosage-information

Chapter 11

Stress Quotes, http://www.brainyquote.com/quotes/keywords/stress.html

How To Reduce MS Stress, http://www.sharecare.com/health/multiple-sclerosis-ms/health-guide/live-better-multiple-sclerosis-ms/meditation-to-reduce-ms-stress-video

Moninger, Jeanette, 10 Relaxation Techniques That Zap Stress Fast, http://www.webmd.com/balance/guide/blissing-out-10-relaxation-techniques-reduce-stress-spot

Chris1976, Transcendental Meditation – Reduced Stress, Reduced Risks, http://www.overcomingmultiplesclerosis.org/Community/Forum/viewtopic.php?f=4&t=4369

Meditation: A Simple, Fast Way To Reduce Stress, http://www.cnn.com/HEALTH/library/meditation/HQ01070.html

Mayo Clinic Staff, Tai Chi: A Gentle Way To Fight Stress, http://www.mayoclinic.org/healthy-living/stress-management/in-depth/tai-chi/art-20045184

Scott, Elizabeth, The Benefits Of Yoga For Stress Management, http://stress.about.com/od/tensiontamers/p/profileyoga.htm

Seliger, Susan, Yoga For Stress Management, http://www.webmd.com/fitness-exercise/features/yoga-for-stress-management

Williams, Ray, B, Do Self Affirmations Work? A Revisit, http://www.psychologytoday.com/blog/wired-success/201305/do-self-affirmations-work-revisit

DeNoon, Daniel, J, Study: Stress Bad For MS, http://www.webmd.com/multiple-sclerosis/news/20040318/study-stress-bad-for-ms

Emrich, Lisa, Stress And MS: The Mind-Body Connection, http://www.healthcentral.com/multiple-sclerosis/c/19065/156041/stress/

Burtchell, Jeri, Study Shows That Stress Can Lead To Ms Flare-Ups, http://www.healthline.com/health-news/ms-stress-could-predict-ms-disease-activity-121813

Multiple Sclerosis And Stress Management, http://www.msactivesource.com/ms-stress-management.xml

Stress, http://www.msfocus.org/stress.aspx

Svoboda, Elizabeth, Beat Your Stress Hormone, http://www.prevention.com/mind-body/emotional-health/how-lower-cortisol-manage-stress?page=2

Want To Sleep Better? First, Reduce Your Cortisol Levels Then Follow These Six Key Tips, http://bodyecology.com/articles/reduce_your_cortisol_levels.php#.U9suAfmSySo

Emrich, Lisa, Rewire Your Brain For Optimism: MS And Positive Thinking, http://www.healthcentral.com/multiple-sclerosis/c/19065/153627/rewire/

Mayo Clinic Staff, Social Support: Tap This Tool To Beat Stress, http://www.mayoclinic.org/healthy-living/stress-management/in-depth/social-support/art-20044445

Chapter 12

Deep Meaningful Quotes About Life For Inspired Living, http://www.healthyyounaturally.com/edu/deep_and_meaningful_quotes.htm

Multiple Sclerosis And Exercise, http://www.webmd.com/multiple-sclerosis/guide/multiple-sclerosis-exercise

Exercise, http://www.mssociety.org.uk/what-is-ms/treatments-and-therapies/exercise

MS and Exercise, http://www.tysabri.com/ms-and-exercise.xml

Exercising With Multiple Sclerosis, http://www.activemsers.org/exercisesstretches/tipsexercisingwithms.html

Exercise and MS, http://msrrtc.washington.edu/info/factsheets/exercise

Study Finds Aerobic Exercise Improves Memory, Brain Function and Physical Fitness, http://www.brainhealth.utdallas.edu/blog_page/study-finds-aerobic-exercise-improves-memory-brain-function-and-physical-fi

Multiple Sclerosis and Exercise, http://www.webmd.com/multiple-sclerosis/guide/multiple-sclerosis-exercise

Understanding MS and Exercise: A Fitness Lifestyle Providers Guide, http://mssociety.ca/alberta/pdf/Active/UnderstandingMSandExercise.pdf

Pietrangelo, Ann, Open Swim: Multiple Sclerosis Water Therapy, http://www.healthline.com/health/multiple-water-therapy

Kileff, Joanna, Aerobic Exercise For People With Multiple Sclerosis, http://www.mstrust.org.uk/professionals/information/wayahead/articles/08022004_03.jsp

Finding Another Sport To Love, http://www.nationalmssociety.org/Living-Well-With-MS/Health-Wellness/Travel-and-Recreation/Finding-Another-Sport-to-Love

Chapter 13

Sunlight And Vitamin D, http://www.overcomingmultiplesclerosis.org/Recovery-Program/Sunlight-and-Vitamin-D/

New Study Shows Relationship Between Sun Exposure And Multiple

Sclerosis In Norway And Italy, https://www.vitamindcouncil.org/vitamin-d-news/new-study-shows-relationship-between-sun-exposure-and-multiple-sclerosis-in-norway-and-italy/

Stachowiak, Julie, Ph.D, Vitamin B12 And Multiple Sclerosis, http://ms.about.com/od/livingwellwithms/a/vitamin_b12.htm

Wahls, Terry, Dr Wahl's Super-Nutrient Paleo Diet, That Reversed Her Multiple Sclerosis, http://paleozonenutrition.com/2012/02/08/a-new-experiment-dr-wahls-super-nutrient-paleo-diet-9-cups-veggies-a-day/

Williams, Andy, Can Multiple Sclerosis Be Reversed By Diet? http://juicingtherainbow.com/1735/news/can-multiple-sclerosis-be-reversed-by-diet/

Reinberg, Steven, Vitamin D May Slow Multiple Sclerosis: Study, http://www.webmd.com/multiple-sclerosis/news/20140120/vitamin-d-may-slow-multiple-sclerosis-study-suggests

Other Supplements, http://www.overcomingmultiplesclerosis.org/Recovery-Program/Supplements/Other-Supplements/

Multiple Sclerosis (MS) Symptom Treatment With Medical Marijuana, http://www.medicalmarijuana.net/uses-and-treatments/multiple-sclerosis/

Multiple Sclerosis, Four Disease Courses Have Been Identified In MS, http://www.lef.org/protocols/neurological/multiple_sclerosis_02.htm

Vitamins, Minerals, And Supplements, http://multiplesclerosis.net/natural-remedies/vitamins-supplements/

Scheer, Roddy, Moss, Doug, Dirt Poor: Have Fruits And Vegetables Become Less Nutritious? http://www.scientificamerican.com/article/soil-depletion-and-nutrition-loss/

Kempston, Megan, 9 Spices With Super-Healing Powers, http://www.caring.com/articles/spices-with-healing-powers

Chapter 14

Deep Meaningful Quotes About Life For Inspired Living, http://www.healthyyounaturally.com/edu/deep_and_meaningful_quotes.htm

Multiple Sclerosis: Jack Osborne And 12 Other Famous People Touched By The Disease, http://www.huffingtonpost.com/2012/06/18/multiple-sclerosis-celebrities_n_1606174.html

Jack Osborne's Life-Changing Diagnosis, http://www.doctoroz.com/episode/jack-osbournes-life-changing-diagnosis

Multiple Sclerosis: Montel Williams And MS (Contd.), http://www.medicinenet.com/script/main/art.asp?articlekey=53785&page=3

Bloudoff-Indelicato, Mollie, Montel-Williams' MS Routine: A Juice Diet And Regular Exercise, http://www.everydayhealth.com/multiple-sclerosis/living-well-with-montel-williams.aspx

Peterson, Hayley, 'It's A Reminder That I Can't Keep Up The Pace': Ann Romney Opens Up About Her Battle With Multiple Sclerosis During Campaign Stop, http://www.dailymail.co.uk/news/article-2221058/Ann-Romney-opens-struggle-Multiple-Sclerosis.html

Barclay, Rachel, How Ann Romney Tackled Her Multiple Sclerosis – A Fateful Diagnosis, http://www.healthline.com/health-slideshow/ann-romney-multiple-sclerosis#promoSlide

Wilson, Jacque, NASCAR Driver Trevor Bayne Diagnosed With Multiple Sclerosis, http://www.cnn.com/2013/11/12/health/trevor-bayne-multiple-sclerosis/

Trevor Bayne Has Multiple Sclerosis, http://espn.go.com/racing/nascar/cup/story/_/id/9964490/trevor-bayne-says-multiple-sclerosis-plans-continue-racing

Richard Cohen On Why His Multiple Sclerosis Didn't Make Him A Victim, http://www.huffingtonpost.com/2014/01/20/richard-cohen-multiple-sclerosis_n_4632001.html

Flam, Lisa, Richard Cohen: MS Trial May Offer 'Some Kind Of Hope', http://www.today.com/health/richard-cohen-ms-trial-may-offer-some-kind-hope-2D79695844

Cartel, Mari, How Clay Walker Manages Symptoms Of Multiple Sclerosis, http://www.lifescript.com/health/centers/multiple_sclerosis/articles/how_clay_walker_manages_symptoms_of_multiple_sclerosis.aspx

Walker, Clay, Country Star Clay Walker On Living With MS, http://www.cnn.com/2013/02/07/health/human-factor-walker/

Meet Tamia Washington Hill – She And Husband Grant Hill Open Up About MS On EXTRA, http://staging.nationalmssociety.org/online-community/personal-stories/tamia/index.aspx

Tamia Hill, http://www.rateadrug.com/Slide-Famous-People-with-multiple-sclerosis--Tamia-Hill.aspx

Squiggy Has Multiple Sclerosis, http://www.msstrength.com/squiggy-has-multiple-sclerosis/comment-page-1/

Roland, Tom, Ketchum Takes A Healthy Approach, http://www.mult-sclerosis.org/news/Jun2003/MoreonHalKetchum.html

McDaniel, Randy, Whatever Happened To Hal Ketchum, http://kxrb.com/whatever-happened-to-hal-ketchum/

Chapter 15

Quotes About Inspirational Life, http://www.goodreads.com/quotes/tag/inspirational-life

Treatment, http://www.multiplesclerosis.com/us/treatment.php

Hall, Susan, D, Biometric Bracelet Could Send Remote-Monitoring Data To EHRS, http://www.fiercehealthit.com/story/biometric-bracelet-could-send-remote-monitoring-data-ehrs/2012-08-09

Background Facts: Bee Sting Therapy And MS, http://health.howstuffworks.com/medicine/tests-treatment/bee-sting-therapy-and-ms.htm

Kalb, Rosalind, Giesser, Barbara, Costello, Kathleen, Multiple Sclerosis: Establish A Pattern Of Routine Care, http://www.dummies.com/how-to/content/multiple-sclerosis-establish-a-pattern-of-routine-.html

The Woman Who Cured Multiple Sclerosis, https://medium.com/cured-disease-naturally/the-woman-who-cured-multiple-sclerosis-11d2ebe47162

Make The Most Of Your Doctor Visits, http://www.nationalmssociety.org/Treating-MS/Comprehensive-Care/Make-the-Most-of-Your-Doctor-Visits

Shaw, Gina, Treat And Prevent A Multiple Sclerosis Flare-Up, http://www.webmd.com/multiple-sclerosis/features/flare-ups

Madell, Robin, What Is A Multiple Sclerosis Exacerbation? http://www.healthline.com/health/multiple-sclerosis/exacerbation-ms-attack#WorseningSymptoms1

Holland, Kimberley, Multiple Sclerosis Support Groups, http://www.healthline.com/health-slideshow/multiple-sclerosis-support-groups

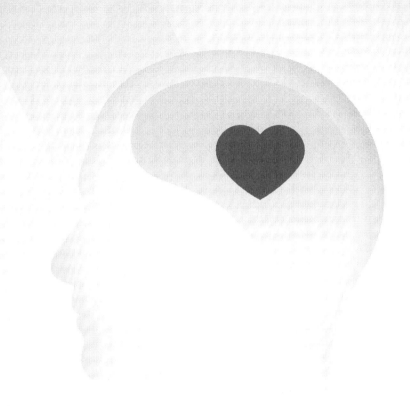

Index

A

Acta Neurologica Scandinavica 122
Acupuncture 68
Adams, Mike 89
Aerobic Exercise 165, 167, 234
Albert Einstein 33
alternative treatments 15, 17, 49, 145, 213
American Academy of Neurology 28
American Society for Microbiology 28
A negative mind 157
antioxidants 68, 69, 130, 177, 180
aqua therapy 170
Ashton Embry 106, 128
asthma 22
Athetosis 39
Atkins diet 115
autoimmune diseases 21, 22, 109, 122, 129, 177, 183
autopsy plaques 23
Ayurvedic medicine 69

B

Bayne, Trevor 190, 191, 236
BBC News Health 123
Bee Sting Therapy 202, 237
Behavioral Medicine Research Center 150
benefits of nutrition 27, 79
Betty Ferber 17
Bladder and bowel trouble 13
Brown, Eleanor 126, 135

C

Candida growth 101
Carbohydrate and sugar detox 132
carpal tunnel syndrome 9
celiac disease 22, 106, 108, 122, 123
Center for Brain Health 165
central nervous system 13, 14, 22, 25, 26, 38, 42, 52, 64, 108, 128, 130, 163, 180
Chief of Anesthesiology, Missouri Baptist Medical Center 8, 245
Chinese herbal medicine 176
chiropractic 54
Chorea 39
clinical research 10, 11
CNS (central nervous system) 22
Coenzyme Q10 180
Cognitive dysfunction with MS 13
Cohen, Richard 191, 192, 236
Consistent Evaluation 207
conventional treatments 15, 16, 52
Copaxone 138, 232
Cortisol Reduction 158
Cultivating a Self-Care Lifestyle 135

D

Dalfampridine 64
David Wolfe 26
Deep brain stimulation 15
Demi Lovato 75
Department of Neurology and Traditional Chinese Medicine in Fujian 176
Depression 13, 43, 156, 157

About the Author

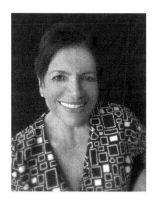

By traditional standards, Cynthia Guy led a life she was not meant to lead. As a 33-year-old Panamanian nurse anesthetist with two small children, Cynthia enrolled in medical school and later immigrated to the United States with kids and husband in tow to practice medicine. She trained as an anesthesiologist at Washington University in St. Louis, Missouri, and doggedly worked her way to becoming Chief of Anesthesiology at Missouri Baptist Hospital, overseeing a team of 42 medical staff. Several years later she used her skills as a medical entrepreneur to establish the first independent pain center in St. Louis. She and her family lived the American dream.

But all of this success did not come without a price—the stress of achievement finally taking its toll in the form of multiple sclerosis diagnosed at the age of 60, which eventually forced her to retire and sell her practice. As an over-achiever, having to slow down, step back, and take a break professionally was painful but necessary with MS as her new challenge. This book shares Cynthia's journey and what she as a physician had to learn in order to heal.

Made in the USA
San Bernardino, CA
20 September 2016